More praise for *Homeopath*

"A book we all need—representing, without any doubt, a ~~~, forward toward possibly defining how Homeopathy works. A very interesting work, about the scientific nature of Homeopathic medicine, written by an excellent clinician.

"Even if it may appear obvious, the first thing that struck me about this book is the Introduction. Sometimes short phrases, often single words, contain a message that conveys specific information in that moment. I think I know Bill enough to be aware of how much he loves Homeopathy and, similar to him, I know many others who are valid Homeopaths and men of science who, with all their intelligence and knowledge, could not and would not leave their skepticism.

"The intention to give serious scientific validation to Homeopathic medicine has been a process in the making for many years, but never has there been such a ferment as in the last few years—fulfilling a great need for most of us.

"Personally, what I often find disappointing is to see, at conferences or meetings, that the only goal is to demonstrate that Homeopathy does work. Infinitesimal dilutions work on insulated cells, on tissues, on laboratory animals, and even on humans. I don't think our problem is to demonstrate just that. I don't believe it to be the principal issue.

"Instead, I think that the task is to venture toward the 'difficult to prove' frontier, toward a reading of the possible functioning of man not only to include the physics perspective but also a vision that integrates philosophy, anthropology, and other traditions—inclusive of everything starting with 'psy' and ending with 'medicine.' Most important is to have the courage to start a fundamental revisitation of how we define human kind and the marvelous correlation existing between man and his medical systems.

continued on next page

"My impression is that Homeopathy in this moment is one among the most seductive medicines to be deeply explored—a medicine in which the link between scientific and humanistic approaches cannot be broken by definition.

"Maybe there is something more—the doubt—that healthy skepticism that made Bill write this very interesting book which surely will add more knowledge and stimulate thinking for us and other men of science.

"As a first wish to Bill, I hope this book will have the great success it deserves.

"My second wish is that he keep cultivating the healthy skepticism his book encourages.

"To be a homeopath means—to wed into One both Knowledge and Mystery."

> —Dott. Massimo Mangialavori Specialista in Scienza
> Dell' Alimentazione, Omeopatia-Dietologia
> and international lecturer

"As a clinician, one can see the effectiveness of homeopathy several times a day. The depth of its action is such that it touches the basic inner disturbance and brings about a quantum leap in the person's physical and psychical state. However, the mechanism of its action has remained an enigma, given that the remedies are diluted to such submolecular levels. Modern science is now trying to find the possible mechanisms, and has come up with some new insights. Dr. Gray's book offers, in nontechnical terminology, a synopsis of the research done along with descriptions of the full homeopathic process itself. I think it is an important contribution to the awareness of the people who dare to know."

> —Rajan Sankaran, international lecturer,
> homeopath,
> and author

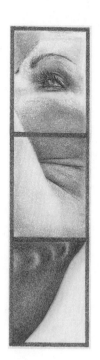

Homeopathy
Science or Myth?

Bill Gray, M.D.

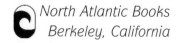

North Atlantic Books
Berkeley, California

Published by
North Atlantic Books
P.O. Box 12327
Berkeley, California 94712

Cover and book design by Tree House Graphics
Cover artist: Victoria L. Gray ("Wesen") Self-Portrait Pencil Drawing

Printed in the United States of America

Homeopathy: Science or Myth? is sponsored by the Society for the Study of Native Arts and Sciences, a nonprofit educational corporation whose goals are to develop an educational and crosscultural perspective linking various scientific, social, and artistic fields; to nurture a holistic view of arts, sciences, humanities, and healing; and to publish and distribute literature on the relationship of mind, body, and nature.

Library of Congress Cataloging-in-Publication Data:

Gray, Bill, Dr.
    Homeopathy—science or myth : modern scientific evidence / by Bill Gray.
    p. cm.
  Includes bibliographical references and index.
ISBN 1-55643-332-8 (trade paper)
  1. Homeopathy—Popular works.   2. Homeopathy—Case studies.   I. Title.
RX72.G73 2000
615.5'32—dc21

                                              99-053966

Dedication

This book is dedicated to my loving, devoted, and patient wife Victoria, who has been enthusiastic throughout.

Table of Contents

Foreword

For most of this century, biological science has been the standard in medicine. Spurred at first by the success of antibiotics, the pharmaceutical industry launched on a quest to find "magic bullets" which would rapidly annihilate the causes of all infectious as well as chronic diseases. During this time, the pharmaceutical and biochemical industry developed increasingly sophisticated methods of synthesizing drugs in an attempt to formulate targeted drugs while simultaneously reducing toxicity. Even in situations in which the germ theory does not apply, as with cancer or autoimmune disorders, the quest for a pharmaceutical based on single factor causation persisted.

For this process of discovery to be effective, fundamental, biological causes and mechanisms of pathology needed to be understood. Science attacked these questions with unparalleled gusto. An entire industry developed into what is known as "scientific medicine." Technology fueled every aspect of the medical care industry from diaagnostics to therapy. This same trend remains evident in the Human Genome Project despite the fact that many geneticists point out that single genomes causing a specific disease will be quite rare while a multiplicity of both genetic and post birth influences will remain most frequent. Concurrently, the information explosion overwhhelmed doctors. No one could master all of it as had been possible in the old days of general practitioners. Specialization became inevitable.

Also inevitable was the cost crisis. Technological breakthroughs, radiotherapy techniques, and costs of developing pharmaceuticals pushed the price of health care to unprecedented levels. As society prospered, health care became a right for all citizens, rather than a privilege of the few. In this evolution, the medical care industry became the largest sector of the economies of most of the industrialized countries in the Western world and constitutes nearly 15% of the GDP of the United States. No other nation on earth spends even double digits for medical care, yet the United States consistently ranks in the bottom quarter of the internationally accepted measure of health. Despite increasing expenditures, the United States position continues to decline steadily since 1960. In short, the United States is spending the most and achieving the least "health" compared to all other postindustrial nations.

In spite of all this progress, chronic disease also thrived as the population grew aged and after infectious diseases were rendered more manageable largely through public health measures prior to antibiotic and other pharmaceutical interventions. Genetics, environment, and lifestyle loom as multifactorial influences on the prevalence of chronic disease. Suddenly, the dream of finding "magic bullets" became increasingly elusive.

Meanwhile, what happened to the patient in all this? Medicine became more and more specialized and as a result more dehumanized. Prevention of illness did not fit in the biotechnological era and consequently received short shrift in funding. Approaches which viewed the person as an integrated whole were relegated to less glamorous and less lucrative corners of the profession.

Public dissatisfaction, however, has grown enormously in recent decades. Common sense led public interest more toward nutrition, exercise, environmental, self care, and lifestyle issues. People are conversant today about "antioxidants" and the benefits of "aerobic/anaerobic cross-training." As awareness grew, patients turned to doctors for answers and frequently found responses lacking in wisdom or sophistication. While remaining respectful of the biotechnological power of medical care when needed in crises, public pressure increasingly demands attention on total health of individuals.

Bookstore shelves bulge with books on the mind/body connection and various approaches toward personal and spiritual growth. Health is seen more as a state of mind and orientation toward altruistic service to others than narcissistic indulgences.

In the context of these changes, "alternative," "complementary," or "integrative" systems of medicine came into focus. People visited acupuncturists, massage therapists, herbalists, and chiropractors in larger numbers than even primary care physicians. Some of these practices are very old, some quite new.

Predictably and appropriately, the response of the biomedical research community has been to seek scientific documentation of the validity of "alternative" practices. Gradually funding is becoming available to research these fields, and results are encouraging. Under pressure from the public and in the face of science, the attitude of doctors is changing at an impressive rate. Medical schools, hospitals, and even insurance programs are implementing and evaluating practices which at first were designated "alternative," then "complementary," and now increasingly as "integrative" medicine. No matter what the terminology, the emphasis is on "evidence-based medeicine" to determine what works and what does not, independently of whether the intervention is alternative or conventional.

Into this arena enters homeopathy. Actually, homeopathy has been prevalent throughout the Western world for two centuries. In many countries, such as France and Germany, it enjoys a popularity equal to that of conventional medicine. Increasingly there are rigorous, clinical research trials, in admittedly limited areas as yet, that tend to confirm rather than refute the decades of homeopathic clinical effectiveness.

A stumbling block to the acceptance of homeopathy, however, has been the difficulty in explaining its mechanism of action. Surely, the extreme dilution of the remedies did not fit into existing scientific paradigms or clinical treatment. Even what scientific evidence has existed in the clinical literature tended to be ignored because the mechanism was difficult to conceptualize. Predominantly, the attitude was: the studies must be flawed because dilutions of remedies go beyond the point of there being even one molecule of substance left! If we cannot determine the mechanism of action, then the studies must be wrong.

Fortunately, Dr. Gray's book addresses that paradox squarely and clearly. In terms easily understood without advanced scientific training, he carries the reader through each demonstration of the evidence. Scientific evaluation of homeopathy has matured in recent years, so this book represents a fresh breeze to those baffled by skeptical challenges.

Research into the mechanism of action of homeopathy actually lies at the frontier of biomedical research in general. Much of what is termed modern or quantum physics is actually based on research and theories that are now over 50 years old. By today's standards, even these reductionistic models are as antiquated as Newtonian physics. In the theoretical domains of string theory, faster than light tachyons, and interdimensional space convolutions, the role of previously inexplicable energy and information systems are emerging with greater clarity to yield possible mechanisms underlying homeopathy. No long polar opposites, conventional medicine and homeopathy are growing closer together and it is a confluence which enriches both approaches.

Bill Gray is eminently qualified to carry this message. Having received his scientific training at Stanford Medical School under the tutelage of five Nobel Prize winners, he courageously took up homeopathy when it was still a butt of misinformed jokes in the United States. he went on to become one of the most vigorous leaders in the rejuvenation of homeopathy as it rode the wave of public interest in alternative medicine in general. His experience as a teacher for many of the prominent teachers of homeopathy today demonstrates the style and clarity of his writing.

Both clinicians and patients can look forward to this volume playing a significant role in the evaluation and acceptance of homeopathy into the exploding field of integrative medicine throughout medical schools, hospitals, board rooms, and legislatures which have become the forums for renewal of the health care industry.

Kenneth Pelletier, MD, Director
Complementary and Alternative Medicine Program
at Stanford (CAMPS)
Clinical Associate Professor of Medicine
Stanford University School of Medicine

Preface

The past few years have seen an astonishing confluence of trends that offer exciting possibilities for those who suffer and the medical industry that serves them. Two centuries ago, Samuel Hahnemann took an ancient medical principle and systematized it according to the scientific revolution of his era. The science he developed worked very well experientially, but research was unable to adequately explain how it worked. Indeed, lack of explanation encouraged those with more skeptical minds who insist on concrete mechanisms to satisfy their beliefs.

Meanwhile, the suffering public in recent decades has been turning increasingly to alternative medicine for care.[Eisenberg DM *et al*, 1993] Indeed, Americans most recently have made 425 million visits/year to alternative practitioners (mostly paying out-of-pocket), 40 million more than were made to primary care physicians—an astonishing fact considering what we call "standard medicine." [Chez AR, Jonas WB, 1997] In lock step with other therapies, homeopathy has undergone a concurrent revival of popularity.

With little fanfare, developments in basic science laboratories around the world independently have generated research that definitively validates clinical observations of homeopathy. Moreover, the tools developed in the course of this research provide opportunities to expand our understanding of the exact mechanisms of not only homeopathic remedies, but of allopathic ones as well.

Throughout 28 years of clinical practice of homeopathy, I have been asked, "What is homeopathy?" "Is it safe?" "How does it work?" "My husband is a skeptic. What science is there?"

It is for that skeptic that I write this book.

An open-minded skepticism is necessary to produce the results seen commonly in homeopathy. Physicians treating suffering people need concrete, visible outcomes rather than mystical speculations. True, there are those who have a bias in favor of traditional methods regardless of evidence. On the other hand, those with an honest spirit of inquiry now have material that can be taken seriously.

Personally, my interest has always been clinical, despite excellent scientific training I received along the way—6 Nobel laureates as teachers. I preferred to leave science to researchers. However, skeptics' questions never seemed to quit. Eventually, delving into the actual research, I was surprised and excited to discover that not only does science validate homeopathy—it now has even evolved to the point of explaining the biophysical mechanisms involved!

There are many introductory books on the market which describe basic principles, practice, and history of homeopathy. There are also numerous self-help books which aid people in treating acute conditions. This book is neither. It is for the skeptic who needs a believable mechanism.

I count myself among the ranks of such skeptics. Indeed, I probably am a homeopath precisely *because* I am a skeptic.

Answers can be delivered through several lenses.

One approach is to deliver anecdotes of impressive cases— examples which cannot be controverted in themselves. Sidebars scattered throughout the early chapters present these cases and some samples of remedy pictures. Nevertheless, a genuine skeptic might dismiss these as merely anecdotal. Where is the real scientific evidence?

Chapter 2 describes in detail double-blind controlled studies on human beings. Chapters 3, 4, and 5 delineate stepwise basic science starting from properties of homeopathically prepared water, to electromagnetic transmission in tissue cultures, and finally to animal experiments. Despite the technical nature of these chapters, an attempt has been made to minimize terminology and mathematics—creating a kind of *Scientific American* version. The information is voluminous, so some readers may prefer to skim some of this material. Regardless, extensive references are provided for those interested in delving deeper into these evolving and dynamic realms of frontier science.

Homeopathy, throughout its 200-year history, has evolved as a classical science based on empirical principles. As such, it described experiences without presuming to know *a priori* the underlying mechanisms. In true empirical fashion, it is database-oriented and holistic from its inception, rather than theoretical or fragmented into reductionistic specialties.

Today, the science is maturing—catching up to its empirical beginnings. Computers render vast databases accessible to review and analysis. Biophysical experiments validate holistic coherence of organisms. New discoveries about quantum electrodynamic properties of water explain both the ultramolecular effects of potentization and the resonance implicit in the Similia Principle. Moreover, science now is focusing on the exact mechanism of transmission of information from remedy to patient.

Chapter 6 is an attempt to describe the subtlety involved in actual homeopathic practice. In Chapter 7, several remedies with accompanying cured cases are synopsized. Thus, homeopathy can be seen as both an art and a science of considerable sophistication.

The final chapter presents some implications of the new research—both for new experimental directions and clinical practice. Furthermore, it is hoped that some holes have been plugged for policy makers dealing with issues of cost-effectiveness and delivery of health care. Armed with renewed validation, homeopathy can take its rightful place amongst mainstream medical specialties.

Acknowledgments

I wish to acknowledge the many researchers who brought about the scientific revolution described in this book. Most of them I have never met personally.

I also wish to thank especially Rachel Gaffny at Rudra Press, who helped immensely in focusing this effort. Thanks to Mitch Fleisher, MD, for the cases he contributed. Dr. Shui-Yin Lo was gracious enough to discuss and review the technicalities of clustered water. And thanks to Michael Quinn for sharing the experience of the Hahnemann Laboratories.

Most of all, I thank my wife Victoria for believing in the value of this project and for contributing her elegance and taste through the artwork on the cover

Introduction

The quest for optimal health has been with mankind since its inception. Theories arose and therapies spread by what worked. Pure empiricism reigned. Often, the functions of healer and spiritual priest were fused, and lore was passed verbally from generation to generation.

The profession of medicine evolved from before Hippocrates based on practical folklore. Eventually, the Rational era came into being. Instead of taking for granted that all things evolved as part of God's Will, early scientists began investigating the Universe to discover laws. Observations became systematized and classified. Basic theories evolved.

As part of the scientific process, the observer and the experiment were separated so as to eliminate subjective bias. What could be observed and documented objectively became the mode of operation. Anatomy, physiology, pathology and other specialties developed. Their evolution depended upon the types of instruments used. Anatomy became histology with the advent of the microscope, and molecular biology became the focus as electron microscopy and sophisticated biochemical techniques evolved.

One of the difficulties inherent in the "scientification" of medicine became reduction of the whole human patient into sub-realms of specialization. Doctors as a profession, who historically were skilled at clinical observation, became more reliant on "objective" laboratory tests. The patient became less of a human being and more of a "case" in the eyes of the profession.

Treatment, too, became more specialized and dependent on technology. Drugs and surgery became more prevalent, while enhancement of health and the body's own mechanisms of healing became de-emphasized. For awhile, especially with the success of the germ theory and the era of antibiotics, the "scientification" of medicine seemed beneficial and rational.

By the 1950s, however, frustration with these trends in medicine began to be felt. In subsequent decades, outright public rebellion has grown. In the 1950s, Adelle Davis and later Paavo Airola introduced the concept that nutrition was scientific, rational, and even necessary for health. The public caught on quickly. Medical schools lagged by a few decades.

In the 1960s and 1970s, the value of exercise became more apparent, and fortunately the embrace of the public led to fitness clubs and the sight of joggers as integral to our lifestyle and culture.

Despite trends toward health, large portions of the population found themselves still suffering from chronic disease. Despite drastic dietary changes, exercise programs, meditation/visualization regimens, and even therapy to address subconscious issues, people still suffered from chronic disease. Granted, statistics improved along with improved health habits, but chronic disease remained stubborn.

It finally began to dawn on people that most so-called "holistic" techniques were certainly *nurturing* to natural body functioning. But what was needed were ways to significantly *stimulate* the body to heal more efficiently. At this point acupuncture became popular and set the stage for the concept that nontoxic therapies might be tried before more toxic therapies became necessary.

On the level of therapy, a plethora of "alternative" or "complementary"—now more appropriately called "integrative"—medicines have developed. Following the lead of the public, the National Institutes of Health and many medical schools, even some hospitals and HMOs, are turning to a variety of nontoxic yet nurturing and curative holistic treatments. The pendulum has swung back a bit from strictly scientific medicine to more empirical "what works" medicine, with a renewed focus on the whole person.

It is in this atmosphere that homeopathy is experiencing a revitalization. Having been in existence for two centuries, the inexpensive, nontoxic, and holistic (individualistic) nature of homeopathic treatment holds great appeal. It is a system based on fundamental, verifiable principles of cure. It can be said to be the epitome of holistic treatment—after having an extensive interview covering all aspects of oneself on mental, emotional, and physical levels, one dose of one remedy in vanishingly small amount is given in order to stimulate the body to heal itself. What could be more holistic than that?

One of the impediments to the growth of homeopathy has been its difficulty in clarifying the mechanism of action of remedies—a problem which is answered directly and fully in this book. Another is the extreme precision, subtlety, and dedication required for homeopathic training—alluded to in Chapter 6.

Brief History of the Spread of Homeopathy

Samuel Hahnemann developed the Principles of Similia and Potentization (described in Chapter 1) as well as many others during his productive lifetime of 88 years. Results in his practice caused patients to flock to him from long distances, especially including royalty of several countries. Most dramatic were his nearly infallible cure rates during epidemics of scarlet fever and cholera.

Homeopathy spread rapidly through Europe as a result of the epidemic outcomes, and soon its effectiveness in chronic disease became clear. Because of its inexpensiveness and lack of toxicity, it spread rapidly to India and South America as well. It was introduced to the United States in 1824.

In the United States, there was meager response on the part of MDs, but it spread explosively via lay people. Eventually many MDs adopted homeopathy wholeheartedly. As a matter of fact, the first national medical association (allopathic or homeopathic) was the American Institute of Homeopathy, founded in 1844. Ironically, the American Medical Association was founded two years later, in part "to stamp out the scourge of homeopathy." [Winston J, 1999]

A remarkable fact is that in 1890, 25% of American MDs were homeopathic MDs. [Winston J, 1999; Ullman D, 1994] The allopathic profession and the pharmaceutical industry were understandably panicked. The policies of the AMA and of most state medical associations were to actively shun any professional or personal contact with known homeopaths. As remedies are given in such small doses with such great effectiveness, the pharmaceutical industry felt very threatened.

By 1911, an economic and political collusion between allopaths and pharmacists resulted in an official report to Congress—the Flexner report—which required all medical schools to have "scientific" laboratories and surgical suites [Winston J,1999; Coulter H, 1982]. This caused closure of all homeopathic schools in the United States except three, which dwindled over the ensuing decade.

Thus, despite continued growth elsewhere in the world, homeopathy went into eclipse in the United States until the late 1970s. The quality of homeopathic training declined over several generations in the United States.

Regardless, a few heroic teachers carried the torch to a new generations of young doctors, who fueled the rejuvenation of homeopathy from the 1970s to the present.

Nevertheless, popularity with the public throughout the world has continued and expanded unabated. Public opinion surveys in Europe recently show that 32% of the French, 34% of the Dutch, and 16% of the British public have reported taking homeopathic remedies [Schulte and Endler (1998) p. 23.] In 1990, 1.8 million American adults had used homeopathy. [Update report, 1994]. Largely, the resurgence of homeopathy rides the wave of public interest in alternative therapies in general. [Eisenberg DM *et al*, 1993; Chez AR and Jonas WB, 1997]

A corresponding interest is occurring at governmental levels in both the U.S. and Europe. Homeopathy has been included in the founding legislation for the Food and Drug Administration. Indeed, the FDA regularly oversees the activities of the Homeopathic Pharmacopoeia Committee and manufacturing and sale of homeopathic remedies [See Chapter 1]. Funding for what is now known as the National Center for Complementary and Alternative Medicine has been exponentially increased as part of the National Institutes of Health—enabling continued funding for homeopathic research.

1

The Principles

Homeopathy is a 200 year-old medical science based on the fundamental principle of actively and powerfully stimulating the body to heal itself. The basic premise is that the human organism—indeed, all organisms—have unique and complex mechanisms to maintain balance. In the midst of constant stresses on physical, emotional, and mental levels, equilibrium is necessary for survival.

Homeopathy's concept of "vital force" is experienced by everyone as life energy itself. It is difficult to quantify, but it is the very real difference that occurs between life and death. Enzymes still function, nerve cells fire—yet there is an energetic change of state.

We all can identify with life energy when we feel happy, excited, and full of love. We also feel an aspect of it when we develop symptoms. Whenever we are stressed or toxified, we feel more limited, weaker, symptomatic in various ways. That, too, represents vital force struggling to re-order itself.

Whatever can be done to nurture the vital force—relaxation techniques, exercise, sleep, detoxification—helps by rendering the vital force more efficient. Homeopathy, on the other hand, seems to directly increase the amount of vital force available. The experience of patients treated with homeopathic remedies is that stresses may come and go as always in life, but the organism's threshold against them raises.

The Principle of Similars

A fundamental difference between homeopathic and allopathic (orthodox) medicine is their attitude toward symptoms. In the homeopathic view—whether on mental, emotional, or physical levels—all symptoms are signs of the body trying to heal. The term "homeopathy" is derived from *homoio-,* which means *similar,* and *-pathos,* which means *suffering.*

The term "allopathy" arises from *allo-,* meaning *other,* and *-pathos* meaning *suffering.* Allopathic medicine considers symptoms as signs of disturbance or alarm. Therefore, the allopathic approach generally manages symptoms by counteracting them—for example, antispasmodics for cramps, antiemetics for vomiting, antidepressants for depression, tranquilizers for anxiety, analgesics for pain. The concept seems to be that disease disappears if symptoms are taken away—a premise that is belied by the emergence of chronic symptoms later.

Homeopaths, on the other hand, observe that mere suppression of symptoms on one level frequently leads to deeper problems in the long run. For example, suppressing eczema with cortisone often leads to asthma. Taking antihypertensives frequently leads to low energy, depression, and sexual dysfunction. These may be considered "side-effects" of drugs, but they frequently persist long after discontinuation. They are not inevitable in the experience of people who are either untreated or treated homeopathically.

The homeopathic approach is to view each person as a whole individual, especially focusing on aspects most unique or peculiar. Correctly prescribed, a homeopathic remedy is designed to strengthen the person as a whole. Symptoms of disease then fall away naturally as the vital force increases.

Throughout history, even before Hippocrates, physicians considered symptoms from two distinct perspectives—the Law of Contraries and the Law of Similars.

Consider a patient complaining of diarrhea. The allopathic physician, by the Law of Contraries, might give Kaopectate or Paregoric to solidify stool and reduce spasm. The homeopathic Law of Similars (*Similia* Principle) would give small amounts of a substance known to cause diarrhea in an otherwise healthy person—thus enabling the process to more efficiently complete itself.

As a further example in chronic disease, the allopathic treatment for colitis is steroids and antispasmodics—to suppress inflammation and counteract spasms. These provide relief and initial remission of symptoms, but do not address the underlying cause. All too frequently, therefore, the disease becomes more chronic and intense, requiring higher doses and more powerful medications.

The homeopathic approach, is to prescribe a substance in small doses which has been proven to stimulate similar symptoms in healthy volunteers on all levels of the organism—not only the cramps and diarrhea, but also mental/emotional symptoms, temperature intolerance, sleep patterns, food cravings, etc. Such remedies might be minute amounts of *Arsenic, Mercury, Cinchona* (from a tree bark), *Lycopodium* (a moss). Each case would get a different remedy, since they are individualized to the whole person. Typically this approach leads to gradual but permanent cure after a short course of treatment.

Thus, the homeopathic Similia Principle states: *A substance which can produce a spectrum of symptoms in a healthy person will cure that same spectrum of symptoms in a sick person.* This may seem counterintuitive to the approach taken by doctors, seen all-too-often on TV commercials, and taught even in grammar schools. It makes more sense, however, when symptoms are viewed as attempts on the part of the body to heal itself.

The homeopathic approach presupposes that the organism is already doing its best, given its limitations of genetics, susceptibility, and stress or toxicity. Somehow, the homeopathic remedy renders that process stronger or more efficient.

Consider the following: All healers, in any culture, survey their universe for substances to aid healing. How is one to know what curative properties belong to, say, aspirin, or penicillin, or herbs from the rain forest?

This quandary was addressed by Samuel Hahnemann in Germany two centuries ago. [Hahnemann S, 1842] Reasoning from the Rational scientific era to which he belonged, he systematically tested suspected medicinal substances by performing ***provings*** in which healthy volunteers took small doses and recorded in writing every minute change—physical, emotional, and mental/spiritual. These writings were compiled into books, cross-referenced by symptom, and now form massive computer databases. The resulting symptom pictures became the basis for matching with the patient's symptom picture.

To this date, homeopathy has a repertoire of over 2500 remedy pictures from provings and cured cases.

Provings can be viewed as a kind of "bioassay" of the healing properties of a substance. Healthy volunteers take a remedy with unknown properties (or placebo in a randomized fashion) and record any symptoms noticed from a previously recorded baseline. The remedy then has subtle effects on the nervous system, immune system, digestive processes, heart, etc. If described in great detail and with an eye to whatever is most peculiar and unique, a picture of the remedy gradually emerges.

Interestingly, some provers in the test group are more sensitive to a given remedy than others. The sensitive one produces very particular and striking symptoms, most especially on the plane of emotions, dreams, and mental perceptions. Other provers produce mostly physical symptoms of a more vague nature.

The proving phenomenon can be seen as an example of

resonance. If a given prover resonates very sensitively to the remedy, the symptom picture that emerges is richer and more individualized. (The concept of resonance will be considered more elaborately in Chapters 3, 4, and 5.)

Consider the patient's side of the Similia equation. Under whatever genetic susceptibility and environmental stress, the patient's system reacts in a unique fashion. Under the same conditions, one patient gets migraines, another hypertension, and third panic attacks. Each has a unique "resonant frequency" or potential which is brought out by causative stresses in life. The full and peculiar picture of the resulting symptoms is what must be "covered" by the remedy picture in order to produce a cure.

In homeopathy, we often talk about matching the remedy picture to the patient's symptom picture. In actual fact, what is being matched is not the "remedy picture" but the picture described by provers under the influence of the remedy.(Figure 1.) I like this way

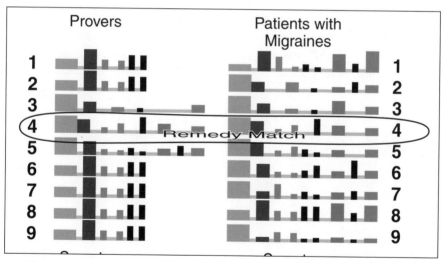

FIGURE 1   Matching "remedy" to patient is really matching the pattern of symptoms (shown as bars here) stimulated in a very sensitive prover (prover #4 of the 9 provers on the left) to a similar pattern in a patient (patient #4 on the right) suffering from migraines. The sensitive prover *resonates* with the patient needing the same remedy. The others match less well.

of describing the process—homeopathy is matching people (provers) to people (patients). The resonance is really between people. By contrast, allopathy frequently relies upon animal studies to determine the effects of drugs, which in the end can only be a crude approximation.

Potentization

The next problem for Samuel Hahnemann was: How can one test poisonous or powerful substances on healthy people—much less administer them to the sick?

After ten years of experimentation, Hahnemann developed a process described as *potentization*—serial dilutions of the original substance interspersed with vigorous shaking. Specifically, an alcohol tincture of the original substance (plant, mineral, animal product) is diluted 1:100. The vial is vigorously shaken (with the force of pounding a leather-bound book) for 40 or so *succussions.* This then is further diluted 1:100 and shaken. And the process continues in kind.

Hahnemann and subsequent homeopaths found empirically an amazing fact—**the more a remedy is shaken and diluted, the**

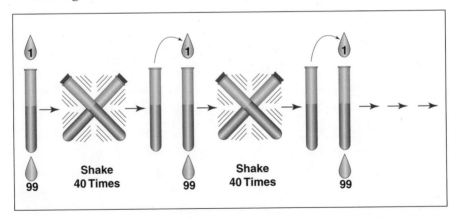

FIGURE 2   The process of "potentization." One drop of original substance is diluted in 99 drops of water. The vial is shaken ("succussed") 40 times. Then one drop of that solution is diluted in another 99 drops of water, the resulting solution is shaken. . . . And the process continues.

more the curative power is increased (provided the choice of remedy is matched accurately by the Similia Principle)—**while simultaneously decreasing toxicity.** [Hahnemann S, 1842]

This observation is truly astonishing when one considers that methods of increasing cure while reducing toxicity have been the Holy Grail of all forms of medicine throughout history! Hahnemann himself probably did not understand *how* this worked. Indeed, the actual mechanism has become clear only in recent years with the advent of quantum electrodynamic research.

Even more astounding is the fact that there seems to be no limit to this. Diluting past the point at which there is no molecule of the original substance left continues to enhance curative power without toxicity! Until now, this seems to defy known laws of chemistry. Chapter 3 will reveal the true mechanism of creation of coherent clusters in water, which does not actually require presence of the original substance.

The Evidence in Cases

Any red-blooded confirmed skeptic has to ask, "How do we know this actually works?"

This is a valid question. The first obvious answer lies in the cases themselves. Classic double-blind controlled studies do exist and are enumerated in the next chapter. For the true clinician—and for most people looking for help—a few cases that cannot be explained by any other means bring the point home more directly than all studies.

Let me describe a few cases from my own experience. Admittedly these are simple, unsophisticated prescriptions, but they illustrate the phenomenon well. More cases, both acute and chronic, are sprinkled throughout the book in sidebars.

A Drowning Victim

Alec [all case names are invented], an energetic seven year-old boy, was diving for something in a school swimming pool. He caught his hand in a faulty drain and drowned. He was pulled out and given artificial respiration, but had suffered massive brain damage. After extensive hospitalization and rehabilitation, Alec had only minimal function. He was unable to speak at all but sometimes seemed to comprehend others. He stared at the TV but showed no signs of understanding. Alec was hand-fed by his dedicated mother and grandmother. Inability to use his limbs caused severe muscular atrophy. His body was so contracted that he could only be carried from place to place—like a beach ball— in his mother's arms.

One day years later, Alec was brought into my office because it seemed to his mother that he had stomach cramps after eating. She hoped homeopathy might help for that at least. I gave *Colocynthis* 200 (made from Cucumber) for the cramps, which did help. A few months later I gave *Arnica* 1M [potency to be explained later].

After the first remedy, not only did his cramps improve but Alec's muscles in general began to relax. He started relating to other people with his eyes. He watched TV as before but now seemed to follow the plot of cartoons. Alec was more animated while eating and even smiled on occasion.

After *Arnica* there were more striking changes month by month. Alec watched TV and laughed openly at cartoons. He related energetically with others and even smiled at me on the first follow-up interview. He slowly became able to feed himself and was able to move his limbs to full extension.

After several months, Alec progressed to walking, and ultimately even to riding his bicycle! Speech came back slowly, and he showed interest in TV and books, eventually going back to school. When tested by the school psychologists, they were amazed to find that Alec tested at about the same level as his peers! It is now about 18 years since I last saw him. To my knowledge, there are no residual impairments at all.

This case is a most dramatic demonstration of the notion that not all cells are necessarily killed in so-called "brain damage." It is known from research on animals that neurons do not regenerate. However, it is clear that in some instances damaged cells are merely shocked into non-function. What is required is a stimulus to re-activate, which is what the remedy apparently provides.

A Blind Doctor

At a homeopathic course I met doctor we'll call Andrew who had been totally blind for 15 years. He was so skilled with his laser-tipped cane that it seemed he was psychic.

Andrew's story was truly tragic. He was driving in bad weather with his wife and two children when he lost control of his car, skidded across the lanes, and catapulted off a high bridge. His wife and two children were killed. Andrew himself spent 10 months in intensive care and hospital rehabilitation from severe facial and head injuries and multiple fractures, not to mention the emotional trauma he suffered. His blindness was total from the time of the accident. He was diagnosed as having brain injury as well as optic nerve damage. There was no surgery offered and no recovery expected.

During casual discussion at the homeopathic conference, we discovered that he never knew to take *Arnica,* so we gave him a 1M potency. Andrew awoke that very night after a vivid dream, looked at the clock, and realized he actually *saw* that the time was 3 a.m.! His vision rapidly recovered thereafter.

Cases like these border on the unbelievable. They defy ordinary medical understanding. Being a skeptic myself, I might wonder about the veracity of the author after reading such cases in a book. However, I personally witnessed these miracles and more like them over the years.

I was fortunate in the first months of my career to do my own informal research study. I was working in an HMO as a regular physician, seeing 50 patients in 12 hour shifts. I had taken a one-month course in homeopathy, so I had basic knowledge. It happened that a very severe influenza struck the nation. The typical case lasted two weeks, with people forced out of work. They came into the HMO to be diagnosed, but after checking for complications all we could do was to suggest aspirin and bedrest and time.

With my meager training, I could still see two homeopathic remedies that could be easily distinguished, so I quietly offered to give them remedies after hours at no charge if they would promise to report back to me. I treated 40 cases, and 37 were completely well in 12–24 hours (rather than the routine 2 weeks)! And the three that were not cured lived in the same house, which reeked of mothballs (a known antidote to remedies).

This experience was enough to convince the clinician in me. After all, this treatment was effective, nontoxic, and relatively inexpensive!

To be sure, the majority of homeopathic cases exhibit gradual improvement over time—perhaps two or more years in chronic conditions on average. So not all stories represent miracles

Placebo Effect?

The proper skeptic is bound to ask further, "How do we know that this isn't just placebo effect?"

I am commonly asked this question, especially during talks before allopathic doctors. My first answer is, "If placebo effect is this effective—and nontoxic—we should all be doing it!" ... Of course, this is not really a satisfying answer.

The woman who drove off a cliff

Early in my medical practice, I was asked by a nurse to see her 20 year-old daughter Pat [no patient names are real in this book] in the hospital. Ten days earlier, after a Saturday night party and considerable alcohol, she misjudged a turn and drove off a cliff. Her car was totalled, and she by all rights should have been killed. She had a severe head injury and multiple bruises, but was thankfully alive.

When I saw Pat in the hospital, she was still pretty banged up. Her forehead was black and blue. Her eyes were swollen nearly shut. There was a ten-inch laceration carefully stitched diagonally across her forehead. She spoke slowly and thickly both because of pain and because of mental dullness.

Pat still had signs of concussion. As she looked at the newspaper in front of her, she could not comprehend the words. It was hard for her to think. She felt "like mush." These are fairly common symptoms in concussion, but it was unusual to experience them so severely ten days later.

Continued on page 17

Undoubtedly there is a lot of placebo effect in homeopathy because homeopaths do listen to the *whole* person. As any physician might, we will encourage placebo effect wherever possible. But it cannot explain the whole story.

Homeopathy does treat infants and animals very effectively. Placebo effect presumably is not operative in such instances. Many of the sidebar stories illustrate this, as do the veterinary researches in Chapters 2, 4, and 5.

FDA and Other Agencies

The Food and Drug Administration (FDA) was created in 1937 by the Food and Drug Act. Homeopathy was still known at that point in time and was generally regarded as safe. Therefore, the Homeopathic Pharmacopoeia was established as the official compendium of standards for preparation of remedies, just as the allopathic pharmacopoeia was for drugs.

The Homeopathic Pharmacopoeia is updated on a regular basis by a conscientious committee of homeopaths and pharmacists who remain in close contact with other official agencies throughout the world.

Continued from page 16

For a homeopath, the decision of which remedy to give was simple: *Arnica montana*. In this case, I gave it in 1M potency. I had a small bottle of it with me. It contained tiny sugar granules saturated with a solution of the remedy. I poured it onto her tongue, and she chewed the little "candies" with a crunching sound.

That was it. No more doses. Just one dose in that moment. I left the hospital expecting to hear from her in a few weeks with a follow-up.

Either the next day or the day after, I was in my office and noticed a rather attractive young woman making an appointment at the front desk. She looked familiar, but I didn't recognize her until I saw the ten-inch scar across her forehead. Pat's forehead and eyes had completely healed! There was no bruising whatsoever! She reported that her mental clarity returned within hours of taking the remedy, enabling her to read a newspaper for the first time in 10 days! She was discharged from the hospital with a clean bill of health and wanted to make an appointment for her general health.

Heart attack

Early in my career, I was covering the local hospital's emergency room. A very drunk Mexican-American farmworker we'll call Manuel came one evening with crushing chest pains and shortness of breath. I admitted him to the Intensive Care Unit immediately because he was blue, sweaty, and shocky. EKG confirmed his myocardial infarction (heart attack), as did a blood test for CPK (creatine phosphokinase), a cardiac enzyme released when heart tissue is damaged. Chest X-ray showed obvious congestive heart failure; his lungs had filled half with fluid.

Because of alcoholism and liver damage, I was reluctant to give cardiac medication right away. The homeopathic symptom picture suggested *Arnica,* so I tried that first—with the concurrence of the chief ICU nurse. This was recorded in the chart. We watched him very closely after giving *Arnica* 200 every 15 minutes for the first hour, then hourly for six hours.

The chest pain, shock, and shortness of breath disappeared immediately, so we continued to avoid standard cardiac medications. Repeat chest X-ray in the morning was read by the radiologist as "being consistent" with the patient having been successfully treated by digitalis; in other words, the fluid in
continued on page 19

As new remedies are developed and described by provings, they are introduced into the Pharmacopoeia and thus accepted by the FDA.

In the face of the growing popularity of homeopathic remedies, the FDA has had to deal with a flood of combination remedies—collections of remedies mixed into the same solution in hope of hitting a few that might be effective. These remedies are prepared homeopathically but not prescribed by homeopathic principles. They are usually labeled as being for "Allergies," "Headaches," "Insomnia," "Menstrual Cramps," etc. The FDA regularly reviews these products and disallows them if labeled for chronic conditions.

In 1972, a landmark study was published in the *New England Journal of Medicine* which demonstrated that the public made more visits to practitioners of alternative medicine than to primary care physicians. [Eisenberg DM, *et al,* 1993] In addition, 65% of people seeing primary care doctors were seeing alternative practitioners such as acupuncturists, chiropractors, homeopaths, and others—without telling their doctors. This sparked interest in the medical profession and led to the establishment of the Office of Alternative Medicine within the National Institutes of Health. The legislation funding this agency has recently been renewed and vastly increased into the National Center for Complementary and Alternative Medicine. This funding has

Continued from page 18

his lungs had disappeared.

Interestingly, this patient did so well that he signed himself out of the hospital "against medical advice" within a few days because I would not allow him to smoke cigarettes in the presence of oxygen!

Two years later he visited me in my office mostly out of gratitude. He had no recurrence of cardiac symptoms, had stopped drinking altogether, and even stopped smoking!

spurred a variety of types of research into the validity of alternative medicine and has helped to legitimize its role.

Pharmaceutical Manufacturing

Since homeopathic prescribing depends on the Similia Principle and potentization, correct preparation and purity are vital.

Provings on healthy volunteers are done using remedies made from specific preparations. For example, *Calcarea carbonica* is one of the most common remedies used throughout history. It is made from an oyster shell collected two centuries ago by Hahnemann off the coast of Germany. Nowadays those seas are contaminated. Would the symptom picture from such an oyster be the same as in Hahnemann's era? It is doubtful. Therefore, a pharmacist and friend of mine, Michael Quinn, sought carefully for an uncontaminated oyster from the general region. I had the privilege of locating a few in a fish market supplied by the protected oyster research farm of the University of Oslo. Following a seminar I gave in Norway, I brought these oysters home to California, where I witnessed Michael's care in scraping out the inner portion of the shell according to detailed

Dog's Tail Caught in a Car Door

This is a personal story. One evening, I was loading our dog into the back seat of our car. He hesitated a bit getting in, and I accidentally slammed the door on his tail—quite hard. Normally stoic, he was yelping loudly, to the point where my poor wife was getting sick in sympathy. I was afraid I had fractured his tail. We got out *Hypericum* 1M and gave it to him. Within seconds he was calm and playful. Even yanking his tail caused no pain whatsoever.

A Personal Hypericum Story

Speaking of *Hypericum,* I recall a personal instance which taught me how quickly remedies can act. I was sitting in a reclining lawn chair and caught my finger in the saw-tooth latching mechanism. I felt excruciating pain shoot from my finger up my arm and almost passed out. I managed to have my brother get me *Hypericum.* Within a literal second of the remedy touching my tongue, the pain miraculously disappeared completely! Truly, there was not even time for it to be absorbed into the blood stream and circulated throughout the body. My conclusion from this personal experience was that remedies act by affecting the energetic field of the body.

descriptions derived from Hahnemann's writings. This then became the basis of *Calcarea carbonica* potencies made by the internationally famous Hahnemann Laboratories in San Rafael, CA.

Such precision in preparation extends to all remedies—whether minerals or metals with chemical purity, or plants which must be grown in certain types of soil, sunlight, and rainfall. Specifications as to which part of the plant is to be used, in which season it is to be collected, and precisely how long and in what type of solvent it is to be macerated and stored in are all standardized by the Homeopathic Pharmacopoeia Committee of the United States.

Since the properties of the original substance (or **solute** as it is termed in chemistry) are potentized by shaking and diluting, it is important to guard against any impurities that might not have been found in the original provings. For this reason, manufacturers have taken exaggerated care to guard against contamination.

As in any profession, some

pharmacies exercise more care than others, so pharmacies through-out the world do in fact differ in effectiveness.

I have been fortunate to have witnessed the origin and growth of the Hahnemann Laboratories. Let me describe a visit to their plant in San Rafael.

First of all, the location of the plant was carefully chosen to avoid as much as possible any contamination from air and water. It is located on the edge of San Rafael, toward the hillside of Marin County, just north of San Francisco.

One cannot merely walk up to the door and enter casually. There is no retail outlet, in order to minimize foot traffic into the plant. For my appointment, Michael met me at the locked door.

The doors swoosh from seals that keep the rooms hermetically sealed and compartmentalized. Air inside the plant is highly filtered

---

Baby who fell downstairs

From Mitch Fleisher, M.D.:

"A.J. was the 6 month old daughter of a small town neighborhood mother of five who lived just across the street from my wife and I, and had brought her to my doorstep late one evening in near hysteria, knowing I was a local doctor who did housecalls. She and her husband had returned home from a rare night out to find that the babysitter had accidentally dropped A.J. down a flight of stairs. The baby appeared listless in her mother's arms, its eyes were rolled back in its head and there was a considerable, bruised knot (3 by 4 cm. Subperiosteal hematoma) over the left upper forehead, as well as a small bruise (3 by 5 mm. Subconjunctival hematoma) over the left eyeball. I immediately rushed to my home pharmacy and then placed a few pellets of *Arnica* 1M under the baby's tongue and, because I was concerned about serious neurological injury, insisted that the parents take her to the nearest ER a.s.a.p., which was about 40 miles away. About a week later, the mom came by to thank me and related that by the time they had gotten A.J. to the ER, which took almost an hour after the dose of *Arnica*, when the ER physician on-duty examined the baby and found no sign of injury, he openly wondered why they travelled so far for nothing. Needless-to-say, we were all amazed and delighted at the incredibly rapid and complete recovery from a potentially serious head trauma after a single dose of *Arnica*.

by very expensive equipment and maintained at a slightly positive pressure so that the air flow is always outward, to keep dust out.

The floors are concrete (steel-reinforced against earthquake possibilities), and the walls are prefabricated modules that can be moved to allow for expansion. They are also easy to wash. Store rooms have racks made of steel, and materials are kept in plastic boxes to minimize dust. The entire interior of the plant is kept so clean and sealed that it seems inconceivable that even an ant could get in.

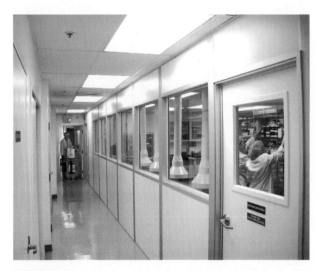

FIGURE 3   Hahnemann Laboratories, San Rafael, CA.

The main work areas have large windows through which the workers can be easily viewed. They wear shoe and hair coverings similar to what might be seen in a surgical suite or a NASA clean room. Formica tabletops and hoods are seen around the periphery.

Extraordinarily, whenever a worker medicates a vial of sugar granules to send to the customer, pharmacy policy requires a second worker to observe. This prevents inadvertent mistakes by distraction or forgetfulness.

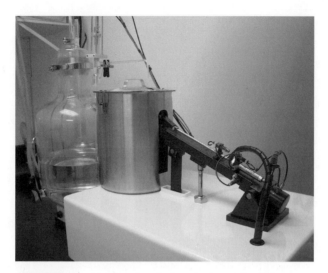

FIGURE 4   Hahnemann Laboratories potentizing machine in extreme NASA-like clean room.

The potentization process itself is done in a separate room by an automated, computer-driven robot device invented by Michael Quinn. A rather loud din of machinery comes from the air-filtering equipment that ensures that the air in the potentization room is as clean as anywhere in the world. The machine's arm holds a test tube which is filled by a jet of double-distilled de-ionized water. The tube is pounded vigorously with a intensity somewhat stronger than the historical "pounding against a leather-bound book" force. The tube's contents are then poured into a basin to prepare for the next injected dilution. The entire process has been carefully calibrated to certify that the degree of dilution is precise.

The number of dilutions and successions are recorded by an automated counter. Once finished, the final potency is poured over sugar granules that are made with chemical-standard purity and enclosed in labeled, brown-glass vials. (This is the step that must be witnessed by another employee.) These are all labeled extremely carefully. Every step in the process is documented in triplicate. Mail orders are received from all over the world, and shipments are made via UPS, Federal Express, and regular mail.

It is known that remedies can be destroyed by excessive heat. Sometimes, the mailed package may sit in a delivery truck or outdoor mailbox that can exceed the 120° that can damage the remedy, so the Hahnemann Laboratories encloses a temperature gauge that turns black and signals the patient to call for another delivery.

The extensive paperwork involved is truly daunting. It is required by FDA standards, which are derived from allopathic pharmaceutical procedures. Many have to do with lot numbers and purity documentation, which makes sense. But they also demand that a diagnosis be put on the label, which is inappropriate because remedies are chosen for the individual, not the diagnosis. Another ridiculous requirement is the "Expiration Date." Remedies last forever if not exposed

---

Near-Death Injury

From Mitch Fleisher, M.D.:

"B.T. was a 36 y.o. carpenter from Alabama who came to my office for homeopathic medical care after all conventional attempts to help him had failed. He had developed a severely and relentlessly painful condition called Reflex Sympathetic Dystrophy Syndrome (RSDS) of his entire right side after a serious, near-death injury sustained while engaged in reclamation work after a major hurricane. He had been cutting fallen trees with a chainsaw when a large trunk stuck under a collapsed wall flung up and struck him in the chest sending him sailing over 30 feet through the air, by eyewitnesses' accounts, landing flat on his back in rubble. His coworkers rushed to his aid, and finding him lifeless, began CPR. B.T., who was a good old Southern boy and not quite the metaphysical type, described his near-death experience quite poignantly. He found himself floating blissfully far above while his buddies worked feverishly to help his battered body. He recalled following the ambulance to the ER and witnessing the hubbub of doctors and nurses frantically administering life support, yet he felt no desire to return to that world. Then, when he was apparently declared dead and CPR was ceased, he saw his wife and children brought by weeping. At that moment, he realized he couldn't leave them yet and, in the next instant, was back in his body with a jolt and

Continued on page 25

to direct sunlight, so there is no "Expiration Date." These labeling problems sometimes cause confusion for patients, but do not affect the power of the remedies—if properly prescribed by the Principle of Similars, of course.

Summary

The first Principle of Homeopathy is that of Similars. *A substance which can produce a spectrum of symptoms in a healthy person can cure that spectrum of symptoms in a sick person.* This can best be understood as a resonance phenomenon in which the remedy of like resonance is capable of stimulating the body to heal itself.

The second principle is that of potentization. The original substance is diluted serially, with vigorous shaking in between. This is

was subsequently successfully resuscitated. Over the eight years since his injury prior to his visit with me, he had taken daily large doses of strong narcotic pain medications, undergone extensive physical therapies and nerve block injections all without relief of his constant, excruciating RSDS pains, which he described as searingly hot thunderbolts shooting down from his right shoulderblade into his right leg which would burn and ache and then leave his leg cold, dead, heavy and useless. He could not sit or lie on his right side due to exacerbation of the pain. B.T., who had been very active and productive prior to his injury, had become very depressed due to his inability to work and frustrated being on total disability. He came to homeopathic care after being told by his doctors that the last resort to possibly relieve his pain was a risky brain surgery that would leave him permanently numb on the right side of his body. Considering his constitutional case, I began his treatment with a dose of *Arnica* 50M to address the initial trauma several years ago. Within three months, he reported that his pain was about 30 to 40% reduced, he was able to dramatically decrease his pain medications and that his depression was lifting. Over the next few years, B.T. required doses of different homeopathic medicines, including *Aconitum, Opium, Stramonium, Sulphur* and *Vipera* to gradually restore his health and vitality. At his latest office visit, he is now fully employed, working 14 hour days as an industrial plant manager, building a new home for his family, and happy and grateful for the miracle of homeopathy."

done beyond the point of there being any molecule of the original substance present, yet potency for healing is increased if properly prescribed by the Principle of Similars.

The first level of belief of any phenomenon is the experience itself. Clinical experience by the doctor, and experiencing cure in one's own body, are most convincing. Very dramatic cures that cannot be explained otherwise, such as a brain-damaged drowning victim and a blind doctor, certainly spark interest for the inquiring mind. Next is the observation that remedies do work in infants and animals, belying the likelihood of placebo effect.

Remedies are prepared by very strict, FDA-controlled standards in ultra-careful manufacturing plants.

The Clinical Evidence

Despite frequent claims of skeptics, there is a significant body of scientific evidence validating the effectiveness of homeopathy, ranging from clinical human trials to animal studies to tissue culture changes. This chapter will cover the most interesting highlights of the clinical evidence.

It is important first to discuss limitations of standard double-blind controlled studies in homeopathy. The "gold standard" approach to research in medicine and biology attempts to control biases which might lead to false results. The principle is that the doctor might influence the outcome by knowing which patient is receiving which treatment, thus inadvertently encouraging a desired outcome. For this reason, research by pharmaceutical companies is generally held at arm's length in medicine.

Traditional research separates patients into a test group and a placebo group (or untreated) group. Outcomes in both groups are compared by statistical analyses to determine if there is a significant difference. To prevent improper selection of more responsive patients into one group, they are randomized. This is all done in a purely objective mathematical fashion. The mathematical calculations are standard throughout all sciences and are usually expressed as a "p" value. Anything <0.05 or so is considered statistically significant; especially, <0.01 is highly significant.

Patients are "blinded" in the sense that they are not told whether they are receiving placebo until the end of the study. Likewise, doctors are "blinded" by not being told which patient is receiving placebo until the end of the study. By "double-blinding" the study the presumption is that the only factor at work is the drug being tested against whatever placebo effect always exists.

A dog hit by a car

A three year-old dog of mixed breed belonging to a patient of mine was hit by a car. The driver kept the comatose dog covered with a blanket overnight. The next morning the dog was unable to walk because of paralysis on one side. *Arnica* 30 was given four times daily for a week, resulting in complete recovery.

This structure poses two primary difficulties for homeopathy.

The first is that homeopathy does not use one single remedy to treat a disease. The entire principle in homeopathy is to use *different* remedies individualized to the patient, not the disease. Nevertheless, this objection can be overcome by comparing methods. The *method* of homeopathy (rather than specific remedies) can be compared to placebo or to other treatments. A drawback of this tactic, however, is that it often requires a larger number of patients to prove the thesis.

A second, and more difficult, problem is that remedy actions must be measured by effects on the *whole* person—the mental and emotional aspects of which are harder to quantify. For example, consider a study in which the homeopathic method is being tested against placebo in arthritis. Some patients will have significant mental/emotional pathology which will need to be cured before the arthritis is to improve.

Eventually physical effects can be quantified, but this may take longer in some patients than in others depending on how much mental/emotional work needs to be done first. Therefore, a homeopathic trial needs adequate time, which is often costly.

With proper care these objections can be overcome. It requires pretty uncomplicated diagnoses, large samples of patients, and lengthy observation. As might be expected, funding for such studies can be hard to acquire in a climate of bias against remedies diluted past the point of any of the original molecule remaining.

Nevertheless, some very provocative studies have been done and have found their way into peer-reviewed scientific journals.

Results in Plastic Surgery

Though anecdotal rather than systematic science, it is interesting to note the interest sparked amongst professionals involved most directly with tissue trauma.

A conference of Plastic Surgeons convened in September 1997 in San Francisco. *Arnica* was discussed prominently as an aid to healing. Patients who took *Arnica* before and after surgery healed noticeably faster than those who did know about the approach. The effect was so definite that the use of *Arnica* significantly boosted the practices of those surgeons who used it. As a result systematic studies were initiated to scientifically evaluate the results.

Childhood diarrhea in Nicaragua

Jennifer Jacobs is a homeopathic MD who also has a Masters in Public Health, qualifying her to do this landmark study: "Treatment of Acute Childhood Diarrhea With Homeopathic Medicine: A Randomized Clinical Trial in Nicaragua" in *Pediatrics*, 1994; **93**: 719–725. [Jacobs J, 1994] It is particularly impressive that the quality of this research was so good that it was accepted for publication after extensive editorial scrutiny.

Acute diarrhea is the leading cause of pediatric morbidity and mortality worldwide. Dr. Jacobs and her staff studied 81 children (age 6 months to 5 years of age) with acute diarrhea in Leon, Nicaragua, in July 1991—treating with standard support of IV fluids and either homeopathic remedies or placebo. The staff were specially trained prior to the study in the most common remedies used for this condition.

Actual remedies were randomized by the pharmacy into identical bottles. Patients took a dose with every liquid stool until the diarrhea stopped. The number of stools and length of time were recorded meticulously. At the end of the study, the groups were unblinded and results were compared by standard statistical methods.

Results were as follows: "The treatment group had a statistically significant (p<0.05) decrease in duration of diarrhea, defined as the number of days until there were less than three unformed stools daily for 2 consecutive days. There was also a significant difference (p<0.05) in the number of stools per day between the two groups after 72 hours of treatment."

Data in this study were striking, well beyond being random chance or any other factor. This represents an excellent protocol for testing the homeopathic method itself. Remedies were properly individualized by homeopathic standards, results were quantified in ways meeting allopathic standards, and the acuteness of the condition allowed proper time for evaluation.

Recovery in alcoholics and addicts

Dr. Susan Garcia-Swain is a homeopathic MD and addiction medicine specialist. The following randomized, double-blind control study was originally presented as a thesis for the Hahnemann College of Homeopathy and is in the process of being published as part of a two-volume textbook on homeopathy and addiction medicine.

Dr. Garcia-Swain ran a large detoxification and recovery center seeing 1250 patients a year. Of these 703 were divided into three groups: one receiving a remedy prescribed individually by Dr. Garcia-Swain, the second receiving placebo (in identical bottles indistinguishable from the remedy by either the patient or Dr. Garcia-Swain), and a third control group receiving no remedy at all.

Remarkably, remedies were administered in one single dose within the first 24 hours of admission for detox! The rest of the treatment followed standard medication and psychotherapeutic methods given to everyone at the treatment center.

After discharge at 30 days, the patient population was followed for 18 months of aftercare, with an exceptional compliance rate of 96%. Their reports of abstinence were recorded and verified by random urine monitoring.

Results showed that the homeopathic group relapse rate was *32%* at 18 months, compared to *68%* for the placebo group and *72%* for the control group, which was highly statistically significant ($p<0.005$). In other words, one dose of the homeopathic remedy at the onset of treatment resulted in an abstinence rate over *twice* that of placebo/untreated groups! Compared to results in similar treatment centers, these are extraordinary for the entire field of addiction medicine.

19 different remedies were used, not because they treat addiction per se but because they were indicated for the individuals.

Otitis Media in Children

A common problem of concern to parents is ear infections and the possible sequela of hearing loss. Clinical experience is uniform in homeopathic practice that otitis media can be treated successfully, without danger of hearing loss. A major difficulty in such a study is its duration.

To answer this issue, the following prospective study was done by Friese *et al.* [Friese KH, 1997] One homeopathic and four conventional ENT practitioners observed 131 children of between 6 months and 11 years of age. The homeopathic group received single remedies *(Aconitum napellus, Apis mellifica, Belladonna, Capsicum, Chamomilla, Kali bichromicum, Lachesis, Lycopodium, Mercurius solubilis, Okouhaka, Pulsatilla, Silica)*, whereas the allopathic group received nose drops, antibiotics, and/or antipyretics. The main

Severe Auto Accident

From Mitch Fleisher, M.D.:

"In July 1991, I received an urgent call from the leader of a homeopathic study group in northern Virginia that one of their nurse members and her family had been in a terrible auto accident. K.L. had sustained serious pelvic fractures, her husband, H.L., was comatose with a severe head injury and their 5 y.o. daughter had been killed, when a drunk driver ran into their car stalled on the side of the highway. H.L. had been working on the engine when the car was struck from behind. The family was rushed to the local University ER where K.L. demanded homeopathic treatment for herself and her husband but was denied it. She refused to take allopathic drugs despite a triple, floating fracture of the pelvis with a large hematoma. She was given repetitive, alternating doses of *Arnica* 1M and *Bellis perennis* 1M for the first few days, followed by *Symphytum* 30C twice daily for two weeks. Though the usual treatment for her fracture is several months of pelvic traction in bed, K.L. was discharged from the hospital within three weeks virtually symptom-free. Her husband was not so fortunate. H.L. was isolated in the neurosurgical ICU in critical condition, and was prevented from receiving homeopathic treatment initially. The neurosurgical team had put him on an experimental I.V. drug for brain swelling, but without the family's written consent. After several hours on the allopathic drug, he continued to deteriorate so his doctors decided to curtail further treatment in the belief that his case was hopeless and terminal. It was a surreal scene; he was hooked up to several beeping monitors which revealed weakening vital signs. H.L. was given only a few hours to live; he was in a deep coma, unresponsive to painful stimuli. It was at that point that K.L.'s nurse colleagues from the homeopathic study group were able to gain access to H.L. in the ICU and give remedies. Contemplating the severity of his condition, my clinical intuition told me to give H.L. a combination of *Arnica* 10M and *Hypericum* 1M, in liquid form, for brain and spinal trauma. The homeopathic nurse administered a few drops on his tongue every 15 minutes as instructed. Soon after the sixth dose, H.L. suddenly opened his eyes wide with fright and sat partially up in bed, startling his caregivers, and then drifted back into a stupor. After several more doses, his vital signs gradually stabilized and he came out of the coma into a deep, snoring sleep state, now responsive to pain and voice stimuli. Over the course of the next week, H.L. was able to regain consciousness after a few doses of *Opium* 1M. He was then well enough to be transferred to a regular hospital room where rehabilitation therapy, including acupuncture, was begun. He required a single dose of *Stramonium* 30C to cure a residual, one-sided spastic paralysis of the right arm accompanied by convulsions of the affected limb, in which he would suddenly lash out violently with his paralyzed arm, as if with rage, especially when his urinary catheter was manipulated. After discharge from the hospital, he subsequently received his constitutional homeopathic remedy, *Sulphur,* which accelerated his recovery. Despite all the negative, gloomy prognostications given him by his allopathic doctors each step along the way during his prolonged hospital stay, e.g., that he would be a "vegetable" and never function in society again, H.L. made a slow and steady recovery and is now living at home with his wife and children, able to care for himself though partially handicapped, i.e., he speaks slowly and uses a wheelchair, and enjoys his career in computer programming."

outcome measures were duration of pain, duration of fever, and the number of recurrences after one year. Secondary measures were improvement after 3 hours, audiometry and tympanometry, and necessity for additional therapy.

For duration of fever, the median was 4 days in the homeopathic group and 10 days in the allopathic group. Relief from pain itself was 2 days for the homeopathic group, and 3 days for the allopathic group.

Recurrences were reported for one year. **The homeopathic group showed 70.7% free of recurrences, while 29.3% had a maximum of 3 occurrences. The allopathic group 56.5% were free of recurrences, and 43.5% had a maximum of 6 recurrences.** No permanent sequelae were noted in either group.

Mustard Gas in World War II

One of the earliest studies of quality reported in the homeopathic literature was sponsored by the British government during World War II. [Paterson, 1944; Scofield, 1984] Volunteers allowed skin burns to be produced using azotized mustard gas, a common chemical agent used during the war. *Mustard gas* 30c was used **as a preventive and considerably prevented severity.** In addition, after the burns were produced in some volunteers, *Rhus toxicodendron* (poison ivy) 30c and *Kali bichromicum* (bichromate of potassium) 30c were given **as therapy, again with striking results**.

The study was conducted independently in both London and Glasgow with similar results. In both cases, a double-blind placebo-controlled design was used.

Migraines

Migraines is one arena in which homeopathy traditionally shines. An important study demonstrating its effectiveness was conducted by Brigo and coworkers [Brigo 1987, 1991]. Slightly more than 100 patients with migraine had their cases taken in extensive classical homeopathic fashion. 60 patients were selected by the author as

---

Individualized Homeopathic Use

Other sidebar cases describe acute injuries, for which *Arnica* is nearly a specific. But homeopaths also use it when individualized to the uniqueness of the patient. The following extract provides a flavor of the homeopathic literature: "Arnica for Infection" by Deborah Frances, N.D., published in *Simillimum* (Summer 1996, Volume IX No. 2)

. . . I developed a quite serious infection in the soft tissues surrounding my right hip joint, following a small cut on my right ankle that had gotten infected two weeks earlier, and that I thought I had successfully treated with *Hepar Sulphur.* My symptoms at the time included chills with a desire for ice cold water (unusual for me), some fever and night sweats, as well as quite intense pain on the slightest motion. I took *Pyrogen* in a 6c potency frequently, with the result that I was nearly pain-free and generally much better within 8 to 12 hours. I continued the *Pyrogen* for another day or two until it stopped working. At that time I was left with continuing low-grade fever and night sweats, but my energy was much improved, and the only pain I had left was a deep aching in the soft tissues at the site of infection. Recalling my recent reading of Boericke, I began *Arnica* in a 30c potency, repeated frequently, with excellent results. The infection cleared up completely. Since then, I've used *Arnica* for treating infections when symptoms suggest it might be the remedy, and—while it's not a remedy I use often for infection—it is one that I've learned to keep in the back of my mind.

Deborah Frances' *Simillimum* **CASE #1:**

CC, a 30 year-old woman, was being treated with *Arsenicum* 1M for severe anxiety and panic. Her history included a former husband who had been violent with her in their marriage, and had recently returned to the area. *Arsenicum* had helped her greatly; however, it did not seem to address her symptoms of chronic interstitial cystitis, (which I suspect, had she remained in treatment, would have eventually required *Staphisagria*). She stated that her chronic symptoms included mild frequency and urgency of urination, with no real modalities. During the several months that she consulted me, CC did have one acute exacerbation of cystitis, at which time she reported an increase in urgency with urethral irritation (1) [parentheses signify strength of the symptom on a scale of 1 to 3] and a tender, bruised sensation (3) in the bladder. She also reported spasms in her bladder (3) and a sensation of fullness that came and went with no real pattern. There were no other symptoms, and a urinalysis showed only a pH of 7.5 and a trace of occult blood. (Urinalysis is often negative in cases of interstititial cystitis, even in acute flare-ups.) the patient was extremely uncomfortable, so I prescribed *Arnica* 200c every 12 hours, as needed—basing my choice of remedies on her strongest symptom, which was the bruised sensation in the bladder.

Two days later, the patient called and reported that she had had immediate relief of symptoms with the first dose, and a complete alleviation of all her acute symptoms with a second dose 12 hours later.

having a greater chance of a curative response based on known homeopathic remedy pictures. At that point, the patients were randomized double-blinded, 30 to the treatment group and the other 30 to the placebo group. Neither the patients nor the homeopath knew which was being administered.

The remedies used were *Belladonna* (Deadly Nightshade), *Gelsemium* (Yellow Jasmine), *Ignatia* (St. Ignatius' Bean), *Cyclamen* (Sowbread), *Lachesis* (venom of the Bushmaster snake), *Natrum muriaticum* (sodium chloride, or table salt), *Silica* (silica), or *Sulphur*. The potencies used were all 30c.

The patients periodically filled out a questionnaire on the frequency, intensity, and characteristics of the pain symptoms. After the duration of the experiment ended, results were compared and

---

Deborah Frances' *Simillimum* **CASE #2:**

JA, a 40 year-old woman with chronic interstitial cystitis, first came to me in the acute state. She reported that her chronic symptoms included a vague sensation of fullness in the bladder, and some frequency of urination. The symptoms had come on gradually over a few months, and this was the first time they had really progressed to acute symptomatology. Urinalysis, a few weeks earlier, had been negative (again, typical of interstitial cystitis). At the time of the visit, she reported an increased sensation of fullness, but the predominant symptom was a **deep aching and bruised sensation in the bladder (2) and right flank area (3).** She also reported low-grade fever (100 degrees F., orally) and chills, and a kind of **"dazed" feeling—"like I'm not quite there."** She did report general achiness when experiencing the fever, but again no real modalities. She also said she felt a sensation of "jabbing, like a thousand little needles stabbing" in her bladder, but that this symptom was not as significant as the aching bruised sensation in the bladder and kidney area. (A urinalysis done at the time of these acute symptoms was negative).

Since the predominant symptom was this bruised, achy feeling combined with the mental symptom of feeling dazed and not quite there, I decided to give *Arnica* 200c. Within 24 hours, the fever and chills and acute symptoms were completely gone, and she was left with only the chronic vague sensation of fullness and occasional irregular frequency.

---

found to **be distinctly and significantly better in the homeopathic group compared to placebo.**

On account of the careful design of the experimental protocol, this study has been praised in both the homeopathic and non-homeopathic literature as overcoming the usual difficulties in homeopathic research. [Hornung 1991].

Dental Neuralgic Pain

A double-blind study evaluated response to pain in tooth extraction and subsequent neuralgic pain. As the response to such a procedure is rather uniform amongst all individuals, it is possibly to use the same remedies without violated homeopathic principles. *Arnica mon-*

> **Deborah Frances' *Simillimum* Conclusion:**
>
> . . . in the the handful of cases of infection for which I have prescribed *Arnica*, the theme of trauma—recent or remote—presents itself. Although at times its presentation has been subtle, I find it interesting that in cases in which I could not trace the present infection to any physical injury, there was a history of significant physical or psychological violence or trauma. JA, the second case of interstitial cystitis, was in the process of divorcing a man who had been quite violent with her emotionally, and had come close to being physically violent with her as their marriage was terminating.

tana (Mountain Daisy) 7c and *Hypericum* (the now famous St. John's Wort) 15c were prescribed alternately at 4 hourly intervals to 30 patients. 30 others were randomly given placebo.

As many as 76% of the patients treated homeopathically experienced pain relief, compared to only 40% in the placebo group. [Albertini and Goldberg,1986]

Sprained Ankle Pain

A nonclassical combination of remedies was tested in sprained ankles. The preparation was an ointment called *Traumeel,* made of 14 different substances in 2x–6x dilutions. In the original research, **33 patients were treated, and 24 (77%) were pain-free on day 10, whereas on the same day only 13/36 (36%) on placebo had pain relief.** [Zell et al,1988]

The same preparation has been tested more recently in a more elaborate study. The results showed that intra-articular injection of *Traumeel* in patients with traumatic bleeding into joints **significantly reduced healing time as compared with patients injected with placebo.** Assessment was made on the basis of objective parameters such as presence of blood in the synovial fluid, the circumference of the joint, and motility of the joint. [Thiel and Bohro 1991]

Remedies in Childbirth

Homeopathy has long been used in childbirth empirically. Finally a study was done in 1987 to demonstrate its effectiveness over placebo in double-blind fashion. A nonclassical combination of remedies was used in 5c potencies and given twice daily throughout the ninth month of pregnancy. The remedies used were: *Caulophyllum* (Blue Cohosh), *Arnica montana* (Mountain Daisy), *Actea racemosa* (Black Snakeroot), *Pulsatilla* (Windflower), and *Gelsemium* (yellow Jasmine.)

The efficacy of the homeopathic treatment was dramatic: The duration of labor was reduced (5.1 vs 8.5 hours, p<0.001) and the percentage of dystocia (a formal term for "difficult childbirth") (11.3% vs. 40%, p<0.01). [Dorfman et al, 1987]

Another study focussed on *Caulophyllum* 7c alone. it was

Inner experience of a homeopath

Miranda Castro is an excellent homeopath, trained in England. She describes in graphic terms the internal experience of someone trained to identify the specific homeopathic symptoms of *Arnica*. What is interesting is a characteristic known in the homeopathic literature—that people needing *Arnica* tend to be stoic, saying nothing is wrong with them. In addition, this story shows the individualization principle in homeopathy when Miranda took the remedy *Aconite* for fright. Following is her quote from the October 1996 *Homeopathy Today*:

... I just stepped out, in front of a car traveling at about 30 miles per hour. The car ran over one of my feet (and its fender smashed into my leg). I was very shaken and hurt, but I found to my surprise and great relief, that I could stand on my leg and move all the toes of my foot, so I knew that nothing had been broken. The driver of the car (a pharmacist from our local hospital!) was shaken as well, and relieved that I only wanted him to drive me home. I wanted to get at that bottle of *Arnica* ASAP!

I stood in my sitting room and surveyed my state! I was shaking uncontrollably and crying with relief that I was still alive. The words, "I could have died," ran through my mind over and over. Ah-ha! I recognized my old friend *Aconite*. I took a single dose and the shock and trembling melted away immediately.

---

administered during the active phase of labor in a group of healthy mothers (hourly for 4 hours). The **duration of labor,** as defined as the period of cervical dilatation, was **significantly reduced in treated women (227 minutes vs. 314 minutes) as compared to a group of labors retrospectively selected by the same criteria.** [Eid 1993]

The same result was confirmed more recently in a double-blind trial. [Eid 1994]

Miranda Castro, Part 2:

I turned my attention to my foot. It had swelled to twice its size in a short half hour and was incredibly painful. It was starting to go nasty shades of yellow, purple and black in a small area that I knew would spread to the whole foot and up my leg over the next few hours. My shin was also painful and swollen. The pain was intense but more of a deep soreness and this was unusual for me. When I get hurt I usually get sharp or unbearable pains. For example, after dental treatment or if I sprain an ankle, *Arnica* never ever works because I do not have the bruised soreness that guides us to *Arnica* ... and I am never stoical! This time it was different ... I heard myself telling a colleague (over the phone), "I'm OK really, it doesn't hurt that much. It could have been much worse." Yeah, right!

I took *Arnica* in a high potency, because of the severity of the accident and because I wanted results (I was scheduled to be the best woman at my best friend's wedding the following day). The pain eased up within minutes, and I used the return of the pain as a guide as to when I should take my next dose. Initially I took a dose every 15 minutes or so but was soon able to reduce that to every hour or two. The swelling reduced gradually until my foot was back to normal by that evening. The discoloration did not spread but reduced to an area the size of a quarter (and disappeared altogether within a couple of days).

I was also fortunate in that an osteopathic friend of mine passed by my house and gave me an adjustment that helped my body balance from the jar it had received during the injury.

The next day I walked up the aisle easily and my foot fit in those beautiful shoes I had bought especially for the event! The word miracle comes to mind once again. Even I found myself saying, "Well, maybe it wasn't as bad as it looked." Right! A whole (normal sized) car ran over my foot!

Phlebitis during IV Therapy

Intravenous therapy, if prolonged, is almost inevitably complicated by the development of inflamed clots within the veins, commonly called phlebitis. This problem was addressed at the Institute of Surgical Pathology of the University of Catania, Spain, by the administration of *Arnica montana* 5c to patients undergoing prolonged IV therapy. The protocol was double-blind, placebo-controlled.

The results showed that *Arnica* reduced pain, redness and swelling as well as the formation of hematomas (bruises). More objectively, Doppler flowmetering showed an improvement in blood flow in the treated patients. Finally, there was a slight increase in a number of coagulation factors and in platelet aggregation. [Amodeo *et al*, 1988]

Double-Blind Controlled Influenza Study

The following is a surprising study even from the homeopathic point of view. Patients with classic influenza were studied. 237 were given a homeopathic remedy and 241 were assigned placebo in a double-blind controlled fashion. Five cardinal symptoms (especially fever) were followed, and recovery was defined as complete resolution of all five symptoms at 48 hours. **The homeopathic group showed 17.1% recovery and the placebo group 10.3%, which is statistically significant to p<0.03.** [Ferley JP *et al* (1989)]

The remedy used was *Oscillococcinum,* a common over-the-counter remedy used in the early hours of influenza. The paradox here is that only a single remedy was used. Typically, if

---

Comment

Most interesting in Miranda's story is how *Arnica* usually does not work in her system, which typically responds with sharper pains. In this instance, however, the symptoms fit *Arnica,* and it worked. Also, her use of *Aconite* on the keynote symptom of "thoughts of death" illustrates how homeopaths individualize their prescriptions.

chosen individually the cure rate should be in the range of 90%. However, for the sake of this study it was still possible to demonstrate statistical significance with even a single remedy.

Hay Fever

Another study using a single preparation—Mixed Grasses 30c—as an isopathic remedy showed effectiveness in hay fever. [Reilly DT, 1986]

In this study, 144 patients with active hay fever were given a homeopathically-prepared combination of mixed grasses. Technically, this study tested *isopathy* (giving the *same* substance) rather than homeopathy, but it minimizes the difficulties of individualized treatment.

Patients were randomized and given either remedy or placebo in a double-blinded fashion. Their response was measured by standardized symptom scores kept by both patient and doctor. **Symptoms in the treatment group were reduced significantly compared to those in the placebo group.** These assessments were corrected for pollen count, which enhanced the differences between test and placebo groups once unblinded. **A corollary observation was that the remedy group**

> ### Snapshot: Rhus toxicodendron
>
> Rhus *toxicodendron* (Poison Oak) is known as a fairly common remedy in arthritis characterized with initial stiffness, better after warmed up by motion or heat, and later aggravation from fatigue. A thread permeating the story is **STIFFNESS.** Of course, the arthritic stiffness and modalities are keynotes. But even the mental and emotional plane demonstrates the same effect in an interview or social circumstance—beginning with a stiffness of awareness and expression, warming up in a supportive atmosphere, and finally contracting once again upon fatigue or lack of stimulation.

> ### Snapshot: *Natrum muriaticum*
>
> *Natrum muriaticum,* sodium chloride, or ordinary table salt. Warm-blooded, orderly, obedient, reserved but sensitive person, easily hurting and hurtable, tense in body, with headaches, canker sores, eczema, and a desire for salt...and more. Essence of this remedy is **INNER WOUND WITH HARDENED OUTER ARMOR.**

41

halved the need for antihistamines. All these outcomes were calculated to be statistically significant.

An interesting observation is that there was an initial aggravation of symptoms more often in the remedy group, followed by improvement. Since symptoms are viewed as attempts of the body to heal, this is a common experience after a curative prescription and was verified in this study. It did not occur in the placebo group.

Asthma Study

A nearly identical follow-up study to demonstrate reproducibility was done by the same author of the previous study, this time in asthma: [Reilly DT, 1994]

28 patients with diagnosed allergic asthma, most of them sensitive to house-dust mite, were administered either an oral homeopathic preparation of their principal allergen or identical-appearing placebo. Their conventional care was unaltered. **A daily visual analogue scale (standard procedure of estimating each symptom on a numerical scale) of overall symptom intensity measured the outcome, as did objective measurements of respiratory function and bronchial reactivity to bronchodilators. A quantitative difference was observed within one week and persisted for up to 8 weeks. The statistical significance was true to p<0.003.**

In this report, **a meta-analysis (collation of remedy groups**

Snapshot: *Pulsatilla*

Pulsatilla, the Windflower. Briefly, the symptom picture is one of a mild, yielding, feminine personality whose moods fluctuate easily, who are very people-oriented and pleasing (unless their family is threatened), who suffer from hormonal fluctuations, PMS, wandering headaches, gastrointestinal sensitivity to a variety of particularly rich foods, who are sensitive to heat and sun yet are thirstless They tend to be cheerful in the morning and wilt in the evening. They like gentle exercise and fresh air. This is a human picture that probably fits many people in the reader's acquaintance. But it is not fully understood until the essence of **CHANGEABILITY** is perceived on every level.

and placebo groups as if in one study) of this and two other trials by the same author revealed a statistical significance of p<0.0004! Thus, both effectiveness over placebo and reproducibility were demonstrated convincingly.

In this paper, I personally liked the argument put forward in their discussion:

> "The usual response to the possibility that homoeopathic treatments are effective is to call for a mechanism of action—asking "how?" before asking "if?" is a bad basis for good science when dealing empirically with things that may as yet evade explanation. The speculation which follows should be considered in that light....
>
> For today's science, however, the main barrier to acceptance of homoeopathy is the issue of serially vibrated dilutions that lack any molecules at all of the original substance. Can water or alcohol of fixed biochemical composition encode differing biological information? Using current metaphors, does the chaos-inducing vibration, central to the production of a homoeopathic dilution, encourage biophysically different-like patterns of the diluent, critically dependent upon the starting conditions? Theoretical physicists seem more at ease with such ideas than pharmacologists, considering the possibilities of isotopic stereodiversity, clathrates, or resonance and coherence within water as possible modes of transmission, while other workers are exploring the idea of electromagnetic changes. Nuclear magnetic resonance changes in homoeopathic dilutions have been reported and, if reproducible, may be offering us a glimpse of a future territory.
>
> For now the critical tests remain clinical. Our results lead us to conclude that homoeopathy differs from placebo in an inexplicable but reproducible way."

Snapshot: *Mercurius*

Mercury. A remedy for people with tremors, Parkinson's Disease, septic conditions, perhaps ulcerative colitis, gingivitis, and a variety of other physical conditions. They are irrationally impulsive inside while externally controlled, quick-witted and brash, perspire and salivate easily, have great sensitivity to both heat and cold (even alternating), and generally are worse at night. Here, the essence is INSTABILITY WITH WEAK REACTIVE POWER.

Rheumatoid Arthritis Study

The difficulty in designing studies utilizing proper homeopathic procedures was demonstrated by RG Gibson in a study on Rheumatoid Arthritis. [Gibson RG, 1960] In this study the patients were randomly assigned to two homeopathic and placebo groups. The remedies were prescribed according to homeopathic principles, and a different one was given for each patient. Thus, the *homeopathic system* itself was compared to placebo.

Patients were diagnosed according to standard criteria defined in the allopathic literature. 23 were given remedies and 23 placebo. Both groups were allowed to continue standard anti-inflammatory medications to avoid potential "ethical" problems.

Objective measurements were made via an independent assessor, and the double-blind code was broken 3 months later for comparison of results. A single crossover study was pursued by giving remedies to the members of the placebo group—a double crossover is impossible because homeopathic remedies can continue to act over months to years once given. **Articular index (caliper measured), limbering up time, grip strength, and pain (measured on a visual analog scale) all showed statistically significant differences ($p<0.005$). In addition, 42% of the patients were able to discontinue all allopathic treatment within one year.**

Mastitis in Cows

Perhaps the strongest argument against placebo effect is the action of homeopathic remedies on animals—in this case British dairy cattle. [Day C, 1986]

A herd of pedigree Friesian cows was randomly split into two groups of 41 cows. A nosode of *Streptococcus, Dysgalactiae, Agalactia, E. Coli,* and *Staphylococcus aureus* was given in a 30c potency to the test group, the other receiving placebo delivered to the water trough in coded bottles.

The results are shown in the following table:

	Control Group	Treatment Group
Cases of mastitis	10	1
Average # of Quarters Affected	1.2	1
Average severity	2	1
Average duration, days	4.6	4
% of group affected	25	2.5

FIGURE 5   Treatment of mastitis in Friesian dairy cows.

Meta-Analyses

In the past decade, techniques of statistical analysis have been developed to study across multitudes of studies. The studies vary in quality, and the methods used do not compare with precision from one university to another, or even one country to another. Despite these problems, sophisticated criteria for selection of data and complex mathematics enable conclusions to be drawn with some degree of reliability. The advantage of this approach for homeopathy is that it considers very large numbers of people over wide ranges of situations.

The first such study evaluated 105 randomized double-blind controlled trials that could be interpreted by strict criteria. **Of these 77% showed positive effects of homeopathy, and 23% showed no effect.** The overall conclusion was that there was a positive comparison but that no definite conclusions could be drawn. [Kleijnen J, *et al*, 1991]

More recently, another

> **Snapshot: *Arsenicum***
>
> *Arsenicum album*, white Arsenic, a poison. Multitude of complaints such as gastroenteritis, asthma/allergies, dermatitis, headaches, insomnia, plus great anxiety about everything: health (hypochondriasis), finances, family security, with a need to manipulate others for personal sense of security, fastidiousness, fear of death, along with chilliness or heat of the head with coldness of extremities, thirsty for sips, desires lemons, restlessness especially at night . . . much more. Basically, **INSECURITY IN A HOSTILE WORLD.**

First author (ref)	n	Jadnd/ IV score	Condition	Intervention	Outcome	Odds rato (95% CI)
Bignamini (41)	31	40/64	Anal fissure	Acidum nitricum C9	Improvement	
Allergy						
Reilly (14)	28	100/93	Allergic asthma	Individual nosode C30	VAS improvement (mm)	
Reilly (97)	39	60/50	Pollinosis	Pollen C30	Global assessment patient	
Reilly(9a)	162	100/93	Pollinosis	Pollen C30	VAS improvement (mm)	
Wiesenauer(112)	121	80/79	Pollinosis	Galphimia D4	Improvement ocular symptoms	
Wiesenauer(109)	142	80/79	Pollinosis	Galphimia D6	Improvementocularsymptoms	
Wiesenauer (111)	243	60/86	Pollinosis	Galphimia C2	Improvement ocular symptoms	
Wiesenauer(113)	164	60/79	Pollinosis	Galphimia D4	Improvement ocular symptoms	
Dermatology						
Labrecque (78)	174	80/100	Warts	Thuya C30, Ant. C5, Ac.nitr C7	Disappearance of warts	
Leamsn (79)	34	40/50	Minor burns	Cantharis C200	Pain (area under curve)	
Mossinger (88)	144	40/36	Pyodermia	Hepar sulfuris D4	Days to healing (days)	
Paterson (193)	40	60/64	Skin lesions	Mustard gas C30	Depth of lesion	
Paterson (293)	169	40/57	Skin lesions	Individual treatment	Depth of lesion	
Paterson (393)	22	40/57	Skin lesions	Rhus tox. C30	Depth of lesion	
Paterson (493)	39	40/57	Skin lesions	Mustard gas C30	Depth of lesion	
Schwab (1102)	13	60/71	Dermatoses	(only patients fitting) Sulphur	Predicted reactions on remedy	
Schwab (2102)	16	40/71	Dermatoses	(only patients fitting) Sulphur	Predicted reactions on remedy	

FIGURE 6 The tables on pages 46 through 49 represent metanalysis by different categories. Evaluated by "Odds Ratios" calculated by teams of independent evaluators. An "Odd's Ratio" basically represents the chance that the reported results were due to homeopathic effect, whether positive or negative. The lines flanking the data points are the range of statistical significance.

Forest plot: Odds ratio (95% CI) — Favours placebo / Favours homoeopathy. Scale: 0·1, 1, 10, 100.

First author (ref)	n	Jadad/ IV score	Condition	Intervention	Outcome
Bignamini (41) a	31	40/64	Anal fissure	Acidum nitricum C9	Improvement
Surgery & anaesthesiology					
Albeu (37)	50	40/57	Agitation	Aconite C4	Physician's assessment
Aulagnier (39)	200	40/64	Postoperative ileus	Opium C9, Raph. C9, Arnica C9	Global assessment, patient
Chevrel (51)	96	40/71	Postoperative ileus	Opium C15	Time to first stool (h)
Dorfman (57)	80	40/36	Postoperative ileus	Complex	Patients without pain
Estrangin (60)	97	40/43	Postoperative ileus	Arnica C7, China C7, Pyrog. C5	Time to flatulence c 2 days
Grecho (67)	450	80/88	Postoperative ileus	Opium C15 (+C15, Raph. C5)	Time to first stool (h)
Kaziro (74)	77	60/50	Tooth extraction	Arnica C200	Pain
Kennedy (75)	128	60/57	Preventing complic	Arnica C200	Complications
Løkken (82)	24	80/57	Tooth extraction	Individual treatment in D30	Treatment preference
Michaud (84)	49	0/14	Tooth extraction	Apis C7, Arnica C15	Oedema
Valero (106)	161	80/57	Prev postop infect	Pyrogenium C7	Infections
Valero (106)	102	80/64	Postoperative ileus	Raphanus C7	Time to first stool (h)
Miscellaneous					
Bourgois (43)	29	40/36	Haematomas	Arnica C5	Pain score
Dorfman (56)	39	20/43	Haematomas	Arnica C5	Pain
Campbell (46)	46	40/36	Bruises	Arnica C30	Treatment preference
Ernst (59)	59	40/71	Varicosis	Poikiven (complex)	Pain reduction
Hariveau (68)	66	20/43	Cramps	Cuprum C15	Global assessment
Mokkapatti (85)	85	40/43	Prev conjunctivitis	EuphrasiaC30	Patients with infection
Werk (108)	108	100/57	Overweight	Helianthus tuberosus D1	Body mass index < 26

First author (ref)	n	Jadnd/ IV score	Condltion	Intervention	Outcome	Odds rato (95% CI)
Bignamini (41)	31	40/64	Anal fissure	Acidum nitricum C9	Improvement	
Gastroenterology						
Bignamini (41)	31	40/64	Anal fissure	Acidum nitricum C9	Improvement	
Jacobs (73)	34	60/64	Diarrhoea	Individual treatment in C30	Duration of diarrhoea (days)	
Jacobs (72)	92	100/66	Diarrhoea	Individual treatment in C30	Duration of diarrhoea (days)	
Mossinger (186)	53	20/29	Gastritis	Nux vomica D4	Global assessment, physician	
Mdssinger(286)	16	20/29	Gastritis	Nuxvomica D30	Global assessment, physician	
Ritter(99)	147	40/50	Gastritis	Nuxvomica D4	Global assessment, physician	
Mossinger(90)	14	0/14	Cholesystopathia	AbsinthiumD2	Globalassessment,physician	
Rahlfs(96)	119	40/79	Irritablebowel	AsafoetidaD3	Globalassessment,patient	
Rahlfs (95)	72	40/79	Irritable bowel	Asafoetida D1	Global assessment, patient	
Musculoskeletal complaints						
Bohmer(44)	102	100/100	Sprains	Traumeel(complex)	Globalassessment,patient	
Zell(114)	73	100/100	Sprains	Traumeel(complex)	Jointmovement	
Thiel (104)	80	40/79	Haemarthrosis	Traumeel (complex)	Joint movement	
Mossinger(386)	47	20/29	Cramps	Cuprum D30	Global assessment, physician	
Mossinger(4a6)	34	20/29	Cramps	Cuprum D4	Global assessment, physician	
Mossinger(5a6)	4a	20/29	Cramps	Cuprum D200	Global assessment, physician	
Neurology						
AlbertW (36)	60	20/36	Dental neuralgia	Arnica C7, Hypericum C15	Global assessment, patient	
Brigo (45)	60	40/79	Migraine	Individual treatment in C30	Glonal assessment, patient	
Dexpert (55)	55	20/29	Seasickness	Cocculine (complex)	Global assessment, physician	
Ponti (94)	93	20/50	Seasickness	Nux C2, Cocculus C2, Tab C2	Global assessment, patient	
Master(a3)	36	40/29	Aphasia	Individual treatment	Global assessment, physician	
Savage (100)	40	60/64	Stroke	Arnica C30	Survival	
Savage (101)	40	60/79	Stroke	Arnica M	Survival	

Odds rato (95% CI)

Favours placebo   Favours homoeopathy

Table continued on next page

Obstetrics & gynaecology

Study	n		Condition	Treatment	Outcome
Bekkering (40)	5	60/57	Menopause	Famosan (complex)	Symptom score
Carey(47)	40	40/57	Vaginal discharge	Candida C30	Global assessment, physician
Chapman(50)	10	80/71	Premenstrualsyndr	Individualtreatment	Globalassessment,physician_
Coudert(52)	34	40/64	Childbirth	Caulophyllum C5	Labour pains
Gorman (58)	93	60/71	Childbirth	Complex	Labour pains
Gauthier(65)	24	60/50	Menopausal compl	Lachesis C30	Global assessment, patient
Hofmeyr(70)	122	100/100	Childbirth	ArnicaD6(D30)	Perinealpain
Kubista(77)	119	40/57	Mastodynia	Mastodynon (complex)	Global assessment, physician
Lepaisant (81)	45	60/64	Premenstrual syndr	Folliculinum C9	Global assessment, physician
Ustianowski (105)	200	20/29	Cystitis	Staphisagria C30	Global assessment, physician

URI, asthma & ENT

Study	n		Condition	Treatment	Outcome
Bordes (42)	60	40/57	Cough	Drosetux (complex)	Global assessment, patient
Casanova (49)	300	40/57	URI	Oscillococcinum	Fever on third day ('C)
Davies (53)	36	40/29	Prevention, URI	'Common cold' tablets	Patients with infection
deLange(54)	175	100/100	Recurrent, URI	Individualtreatment	Globalassessment,patient
Ferley(61)	1270	60/79	Prevention,URI	L52(complex)	Patientswithinfection
Ferley(62)	487	60/79	URI	Oscillococcinum	Patients recovered within 48 hs
Heilmann(69)	102	40/43	Prevention,URI	Engystol(complex)	Patientswithinfection
Hourst(71)	41	40/71	URI	ThuyaC9+2Otherremedies	Complaints
Lecocq (80)	60	40/50	URI	L52 (complex)	Global assessment, patient
Mossinger(87)	118	40/50	Pharyngitis	Phytolacca D2	Duration (days)
Mossinger(89)	106	20/43	Running nose	Euphorbium D3	Symptoms
Mossinger (91)	44	20/50	Otitis media	Pulsatilla D2	Global assessment, physician
Nollevaux (92)	200	20/43	Prevention, URI	Mucococcinum 200K	Patientswith infection
Weiser(107)	116	100/79	Chronicsinusitis	Euphorbiumcomp(complex)	Severityscore
Freitas (64)	64	80/79	Asthma	Blatta orientalis C6	Severity score

Rheumatology

Study	n		Condition	Treatment	Outcome
Andrade (38)	44	80/79	Rheumatoid artHritis	Individual treatment	Global assessment physician
Gibson (66)	46	60/64	Rheumatoid arthritis	Individual treatment	Global assessment
Kohler (76)	176	60/43	Rheumatoid arthritis	Rheumaselect (complex)	Predefined responder criteria
Wiesenauer(110)	176	80/79	Rheumatoid arthritis	Rheumaselect (complex)	Predefined respondercriteria
Shipley(103)	36	60/71	Osteoarthritis	Rhustox.D6	Treatmentpreference
Fisher (63)	30	60/71	Fibrositis	Rhus tox. C6	Global assessment
Casanova (48)	60	20/29	Myalgia	Urathone (complex)	Global assessment, patient

meta-analysis was directed by Wayne Jonas, who later became director of what is now known as the National Center for Complementary and Alternative Medicine of the NIH. [Linde K *et al*, 186 clinical
trials were identified and 119 met the methodological inclusion criteria. Of these 119 trials, 89 had sufficient data to analyze statistically. Thus, 10,500 patients were included total. Two independent
reviewers conducted the analyses and assesses the quality of the studies with two scales for internal validity. In the Tables, the results were
tabulated according to "Odds Ratios." Greater than 1.0 indicates
greater than 95% confidence intervals for the effectiveness of homeopathic remedies compared with placebo.

Summary

The highly individualized nature of homeopathic prescribing, especially the fact that each case within a particular disease category
might get a different remedy, presents problems in design protocols
for double-blind placebo-controlled studies. Nevertheless, a number of studies have been accomplished with adequate size and controls to demonstrate high statistical significance.

At the very least, skeptics must admit that the research done
thus far justifies further investigation. Even with the inherent difficulties, homeopathy has proven effective over placebo in a variety
of ailments ranging from childhood diarrhea to addiction to rheumatoid arthritis to migraines.

Having demonstrated its effectiveness, the question remains:
How does homeopathy work?

3

Physics of Potentized Water

Despite the clinical evidence, homeopathy has always been plagued by an inability to describe an exact mechanism of action of its remedies. A nagging question has been : How can a single dose of such a highly dilute substance produce such profound effects in such deep cases? To the reasonable mind, this paradox seems to defy credibility. To clinicians and their patients who experience benefits, the mechanism is academic—empirical evidence is good enough. However, to those steeped in our science-based culture, explanations are vital. Without them, homeopathy will never achieve the mainstream status it deserves.

Fortunately, in just the past few years, exciting basic science advances have occurred in understanding the biophysical properties of water itself. Whether by coincidence or synchronicity, these discoveries directly validate the properties observed in homeopathic potencies. Moreover, they are the frontier of what could be a revolutionary era in medicine, diagnosis, and pharmacodynamics as a whole.

As the story of this research unfolds, first keep in mind the fundamental properties of remedies, known to homeopaths for two centuries. Any model addressing the action of remedies must take into account these features:

1. Each remedy must be highly specific and unique in structure and function to fulfill the Principle of Similars upon which homeopathy is based.
2. Remedies act best in highly dilute form, whether as a liquid or as a liquid applied to sugar granules.
3. Remedies survive cold very well, but temperatures above 120° destroy their activity.
4. Remedies are destroyed by direct exposure to sunlight.
5. Remedies are capable of transmitting their potency to another vessel of normal water, rendering it potentized in turn—a sip from the glass then serves as a dose. Homeopaths call this "plussing" and value it as a procedure to use in the home on weekends when need is acute and remedy supply is sparse.

   Likewise, a few granules of potentized sugar, when added to a vial of unmedicated sugar, renders all the granules in the vial as potent in turn—a process known to homeopaths as "grafting." As a general rule, homeopaths do not rely on "grafting" because pharmacies need to sell product in order to maintain high standards of quality. Nevertheless, the phenomenon exists and needs to be taken into account.
6. Remedies continue to act even in dilutions beyond the point of there being no molecule of the original substance present—Avogadro's number (described in the next section).

For generations, homeopaths have confronted these phenomena with various speculations, but none seemed to explain all the properties of remedies. On one hand, the specificity of these properties strongly suggest a physical mechanism, which belies arguments that homeopathy is elaborate placebo effect. On the other, accounting for all the properties has proven elusive—until recently.

The papers describing the science are loaded with technical jargon and advanced mathematics, but the concepts can be described in simple graphic terms if taken step-by-step. This chapter attempts to develop a kind of *Scientific American* description—hopefully a clear, non-mathematical model that appeals to common sense.

To do so, it is important to focus on details in order to come to a believable conception of the mechanism by which remedies work.

The Paradox of Avogadro's Number

Water is basic to all of life. It comprises 95% of all the molecules in the human body [Schulte and Endler, 1998]—70% by weight [Lo SY, 1998, p.42]. Water is central to all enzymatic activities, chemical reactions, neurotransmissions, immune functions, hormonal interactions, and metabolic functions which drive life itself.

In physics, water historically has been considered a simple collection of water (H_2O) molecules randomly colliding with each other. When a substance is dissolved in water—a "solute" in a "solvent"—it is thought to be randomly and evenly distributed throughout the volume of the solvent. As the solution is diluted, the solute molecules get farther and farther apart in what was once thought to be a uniform, random structure of water. As it turns out, much more happens—especially when the solution is **serially diluted** and **succussed** (vigorously shaken)—as is done in the process of homeopathic potentization.

Before explaining the seeming paradox of homeopathic potentization, it is necessary to explain some basic conventions and terminology used in homeopathy.

By convention, remedies have been made based on scales of 1:10 dilutions and 1:100 dilutions. These dilutions are made serially—that is, for a 1:100 dilution, one drop of the original tincture is made into 99 drops of triple-distilled water. This is succussed. One drop of that dilution is again diluted into 99 drops of water. That is succussed. And the process continues. . . .

By convention the 1:10 scale is designated "x." The 1:100 scale is called "c" potency. A 12x potency means that the original tincture is diluted 1:10 a total of 12 times serially, with forty or so succussions

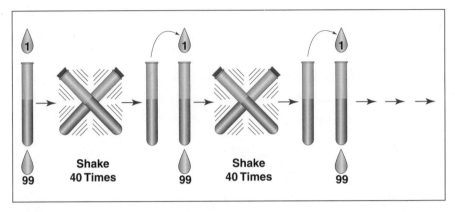

FIGURE 7   Method of potentizing homeopathic remedies.

in between. A 12c means that the original tincture is serially diluted 1:100 a total of 12 times, also with succussions in between.

Because most homeopaths use "c" potencies most often, it is common for the "c" to be dropped. A "200c" is referred to simply as a "200." To further confuse things, a 1,000c (or simply 1,000) is called a 1M for shorthand. The "M" does not refer to a 1:1000 dilution but rather to a 1,000 *c* potency: the tincture is diluted 1:100 for a total of 1,000 times!

Further, we have conventions for even higher potencies. A 50M is diluted 1:100 a total of 50,000 times. A CM potency is diluted 1:100 a total of 100,000 times. A 10MM potency is diluted 1:100 a total of 10,000,000 times. And a CMM potency is diluted 1:100 a total of 100,000,000 times!

Mathematics has a manner of describing these potencies which will prove valuable for later discussion. This is the nomenclature of "exponents." Simply put, a superscript is used to denote the number of times something is diluted, while the base number denotes the dilution ratio. Thus, the designation "10^{-1}" means a 1:10 dilution. 10^{-2} means a 1:100 dilution. The exponent on a base of ten equals the number of zeros in the dilution.

Translating this into potency designations: a 12x potency is a 10^{-12} dilution, which is 1:10 a total of 12 times. A 12*c* potency, on the other hand, is a 10^{-24} dilution, because it is a *1:100* dilution a total of 12 times. By experience and habit, certain potencies are more commonly used in homeopathy. Figure 8 shows the nomenclature.

Common Potencies	Dilution Factor	Number of Dilutions	Exponent Designation
1x	1:10	1	10^{-1}
1c	1:100	1	10^{-2}
3x	1:10	3	10^{-3}
3c	1:100	3	10^{-6}
6x	1:10	6	10^{-6}
6c	1:100	6	10^{-12}
12x	1:10	12	10^{-12}
12c	1:100	12	10^{-24}
30x	1:10	30	10^{-30}
30c	1:100	30	10^{-60}
200	1:100	200	10^{-400}
1M	1:100	1,000	$10^{-2,000}$
10M	1:100	10,000	$10^{-20,000}$
50M	1:100	50,000	$10^{-100,000}$
CM	1:100	100,000	$10^{-200,000}$
MM	1:100	1,000,000	$10^{-2,000,000}$

FIGURE 8   Nomenclature for common potencies used in homeopathic practice, and their respective degrees of dilution.

Hahnemann used quite low potencies early in his career—in the range of 3x to 12x. He was able to treat both acute and chronic diseases with astonishing success. As a matter of fact, epidemics of scarlet fever and cholera made him and homeopathy famous in Europe. This was done primarily with the homeopathic principle and low potencies.

As time went on, Hahnemann experimented with higher and higher potencies. Being an empiricist, he was apparently not particularly dismayed by the phenomenon of increased clinical potency as higher dilutions were used. By the end of his life, he had used at least on occasion potencies ranging to 30c with good success.

Contemporary science of Hahnemann's time was grappling with basic principles in chemistry. The concept of atoms and molecules already had been well-established. And attempts to standardize substances in gas, liquid, and solid form were underway. For the purpose of quantifying chemical reactions, it was important to identify a standard number of molecules which could be compared in relation to different substances. For example, what would be the weight and size of a standard number of gold molecules as opposed to uranium—or for that matter, hydrogen?

Ingenious methods were devised to make these comparisons, resulting in the Periodic Table of Elements, concepts of molecular weights, etc. Most of this was theoretical and at best imprecise until later measurements of electric charge and molecular weight enabled precise comparison.

Pondering this issue, an Italian mathematician named Avogadro published a paper in 1811 hypothesizing an explanation to a puzzling rule of proportional volumes observed in chemical reactions of gases and vapors. When reacting and forming molecules, volumes change in specific ways which are measurable.

Avogadro's hypothesis later became known in chemistry as Avogadro's Law. It states simply that *equal volumes of all gases and vapors at the same temperature and pressure contain the same number of molecules.* In itself, the implications of this law has little meaning in the context of homeopathy. But in chemistry, it pointed to the concept of a standard number of molecules and a standard amount of substance.

Van Nostrand's *Scientific Encyclopedia* (Fifth Edition) defines a generally accepted standard amount of substance. A ***Gram-molecular weight* is that amount of a pure substance having a weight in grams numerically equal to the molecular weight.** One gram-molecular weight (or "Mole," as in "1.0 M") of one substance contains the same number of molecules as a gram-molecular weight of any other substance. This number is called *Avogadro's number*: 6.0220943×10^{23}.

The fact of prime importance to us is that if a gram-molecular weight of substance (generally much larger than the amounts we use in preparing remedies) were the starting point, *the dilution at which no molecule of the original substance persists is 10^{-24}.*

A 10^{-24} dilution is equivalent to a 12c or 24x potency. Therefore, *potencies higher than a 12c or 24x no longer contain even a molecule of the original substance.*

Let me try to put this in some perspective. If we were to dilute *Arnica* to just past Avogadro's number (in current terminology called an "ultramolecular potency"), it would be a 10^{-24} dilution. Put graphically, this would be a dilution of

1/ 1,000,000,000,000,000,000,000,000.
("1 divided by 1 with 24 zeros")

The dog hit by a car whose paralysis was cured by *Arnica* 30 received a potency one million-fold *past* Avogadro's dilution. That would look like this:

1/ 1,000,000,000,000,000,000,000,000,000,000.

The drowning victim, the woman who drove off the cliff and the blind doctor received *Arnica* 1M, which is $10^{-2,000}$, or graphically:

1/100,000,000,000,000,000,000,000,000,000,000,000,000,
000,000,000,000,000,000,000,000,000,000,000,000,000,
000,000,000,000,000,000,000,000,000,000,000,000,000,
000,000,000,000,000,000,000,000,000,000,000,000,000,
000,000,000,000,000,000,000,000,000,000,000,000,000,
000,000,000,000,000,000,000,000,000,000,000,000,000,
000,000,000,000,000,000,000,000,000,000,000,000,000,
000,000,000,000,000,000,000,000,000,000,000,000,000,
000,000,000,000,000,000,000,000,000,000,000,000,000,
000,000,000,000,000,000,000,000,000,000,000,000,000,
000,000,000,000,000,000,000,000,000,000,000,000,000,
000,000,000,000,000,000,000,000,000,000,000,000,000,
000,000,000,000,000,000,000,000,000,000,000,000,000,
000,000,000,000,000,000,000,000,000,000,000,000,000,

000,000,000,000,000,000,000,000,000,000,000,000,000,000,
000,000,000000,000,000,000,000,000,000,000,000,000,000,
000,000,000,000,000,000,000,000,000,000,000,000,000,000,
000,000,000,000,000,000,000,000,000,000,000,000,000,000,
000,000,000,000,000,000,000,000,000,000,000,000,000,000,
000,000,000,000,000,000,000,000,000,000,000,000,000,000,
000,000,000,000,000,000,000,000,000,000,000,000,000,000,
000,000,000,000,000,000,000,000,000,000,000,000,000,000,
000,000,000,000,000,000,000,000,000,000,000,000,000,000,
000,000,000,000,000,000,000,000,000,000,000,000,000,000,
000,000,000,000,000,000,000,000,000,000,000,000,000,000,
000,000,000,000,000,000,000,000,000,000,000,000,000,000,
000,000,000,000,000,000,000,000,000,000,000,000,000,000,
000,000,000,000,000,000,000,000,000,000,000,000,000,000,
000,000,000,000,000,000,000,000,000,000,000,000,000,000,
000,000,000,000,000,000,000,000,000,000,000,000,000,000,
000,000,000,000,000,000,000,000,000,000,000,000,000,000,
000,000,000,000,000,000,000,000,000,000,000,000,000,000,
000,000,000,000,000,000,000,000,000,000,000,000,000,000,
000,000,000,000,000,000,000,000,000,000,000,000,000,000,
000,000,000,000,000,000,000,000,000000,000,000,000,000,
000,000,000,000,000,000,000,000,000,000,000,000,000,000,
000,000,000,000,000,000,000,000,000,000,000,000,000,000,
000,000,000,000,000,000,000,000,000,000,000,000,000,000,
000,000,000,000,000,000,000,000,000,000,000,000,000,000,
000,000,000,000,000,000,000,000,000,000,000,000,000,000,
000,000,000,000,000,000,000,000,000,000,000,000,000,000,
000,000,000,000,000,000,000,000,000,000,000,000,000,000,
000,000,000,000,000,000,000,000,000,000,000,000,000,000,
000,000,000,000,000,000,000,000,000,000,000,000,000,000,
000,000,000,000,000,000,000,000,000,000,000,000,000,000,
000,000,000,000,000,000,000,000,000,000,000,000,000,000,
000,000,000,000,000,000,000.

Count them yourself—2,000 zeros. An extreme dilution indeed!

To the rational skeptic's mind, this information is nearly unbearable. The cases are incontrovertible. Yet the remedies prescribed have nothing in them! It cannot be placebo effect.... It works dramatically even in animals in shock! Besides, homeopathic remedies work only when matched by the Principle of Similars.

So what is going on here?

The Structure of Water

Water is made of two hydrogen atoms (H) and one oxygen atom (O) into a chemically-bonded molecule designated H_2O. As described earlier, pure water is conventionally described as isolated water molecules randomly bumping into each other. To physicists, water has always been difficult to study even though several "anomalies" have been known for a long time—boiling point, specific heat, resistivity, ultraviolet absorption, etc. [Del Giudice E and Preparata G, 1998]

Modern research considers water dynamics as not merely conforming to Newtonian physics, but rather influenced by Quantum Electrodynamics. Newtonian physics historically served very well to explain gross physical behavior, but Einsteinian theories demonstrated the interactions between subatomic forces and field phenomena. Electromagnetic fields clearly affect magnetic or conducting materials, but water has long been considered electromagnetically essentially neutral. This is often almost true for water when viewed in macroscopic terms. However, quantum electrodynamic calculations on the molecular level suggest powerful forces can affect the structure of water.

Simply put, the "isolated" molecules, their motions, and their alignments in space are affected by electromagnetic field energies. Their movements are not always merely random.

To explain this from basics, a hydrogen atom is made up of a proton (heavy, and positively charged) and an orbiting electron (almost no mass, negatively charged).

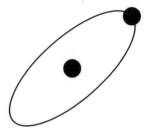

Actually, the electron orbits the proton in 3 dimensional space.

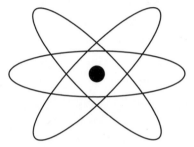

Further, the electron can be viewed more as a cloud around the proton, a relativistic and statistical cloud.

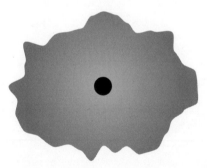

If there are electric charges in the environment, the shape of the electron cloud is deformed by the electrical pull.

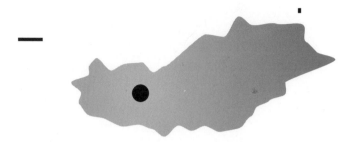

A water molecule H_2O can be viewed as

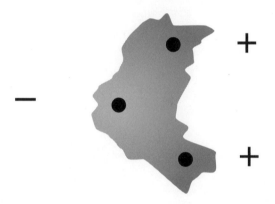

In real life, the shape of the molecules is as fluid as their motions—a very dynamic state, indeed.

For simplicity, let us show water molecules as

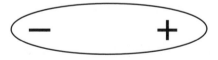

because they have "dipoles" like a magnet.

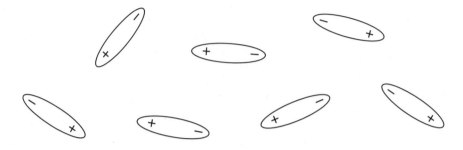

Since like charges repel and opposites attract, the molecules have a weak tendency to line up.

A very fundamental change in the randomness of water occurs when an ion with strong charge is introduced into the solution. Take for example, sodium chloride (Na^+ and Cl^-)

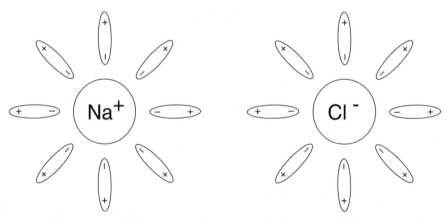

The surrounding water molecules are bound closely in spherical shells around the ions with powerful forces of attraction, similar to magnets along lines of force

In high concentrations of "solute" (strong ions), the spherical shells of water are compact and tight. With concentrations below 10^{-6} "molar" (the concentration of a solution containing one mole of substance), the solutions behave according to chemical and physical principles well-known to scientists.

However, at dilutions greater than 10^{-7} or so, the principles of modern Quantum Electrodynamics begin to take over. The alignment of molecules becomes less compact and spread out over distances, creating regions of "organized" rather than random water. This happens when solutions are both diluted and succussed but not when merely diluted or merely succussed alone. It is in such high dilution regions that pioneering research has begun to unfold.

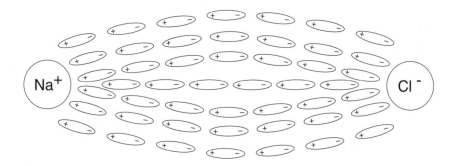

First of all, properties of water with unclear explanations have long been known, including "its negative volume of melting, density maximum at 4° C., and anomalous high melting and boiling temperatures. [Lo, 1998, p. 3] These anomalies cry out for explanations. And such explanations are now slowly forthcoming.

In 1994, George Vithoulkas and his team proposed the concept that Quantum Electrodynamics allows for formation of clusters in water which are bound by forces sufficient to generate further clusters. In their description, an externally applied electromagnetic field fluctuation, or a deliberate contamination (such as a strong ion or charged larger molecule) creates a "local structure" which forms "clathrates"—expanded clusters enclosing smaller clusters inside—which are replications of the original structure and duplicate its specific shape. At that time, spectroscopic techniques had not yet been developed to confirm or deny their model. [Anagnastatos GS, 1994]

In 1988, Del Giudice et al had focussed attention on the concept of *"coherence"—which is defined as molecules moving in a coordinated fashion within electromagnetic waves with well-defined relative phases compared to random water.* The collective movement of molecules in such coherent regions can cause higher polarizability of the water. [Del Giudice 1988, p. 52] The important point in these observations is that "electrical fields can create metastable extended polarization fields in a coherently moving system of water molecules." [Schulte and Endler, 1998, p. 52] These metastable states carry enough energy to be not disrupted by random forces.

Depending on the electromagnetic field and/or the original solute, such regions of stable coherence are specific in structure and vibration. These clusters are capable of carrying complex and subtle information, which matches the requirement of the Principle of Similars basic to homeopathy. Moreover, they are stable and capable of reproducing themselves.

As concentrations of ions increase (so that the ions are closer together, more densely packed), the pressures holding the clusters together diminish compared to the forces between adjacent ions. The cluster "melts" into random regions of water.

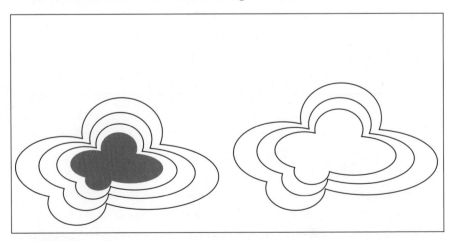

FIGURE 10   Clathrates as conceptualized by Anagnastatos and Vithoulkas.

However, as dilution increases (so that ions move farther apart), forces stabilizing the clusters become more relevant.

In such water preparations, there is a continuous and dynamic process of destruction and growth of organized clusters. In 1996, Lo *et al* demonstrated through ultraviolet absorption (at 190 nm wavelength) that such clusters are stable beyond 10^{-6}M dilutions. [Lo SY, 1996]

A further important observation of Lu et al is that non-ionic substances produced similar clusters. Thus, complex proteins or other components from which remedies are made are capable of creating water clusters. This means that proteins or other complex molecules from herbs or other homeopathic products could be capable of creating clusters. In turn, this is important to the homeopathic Principle of Similars.

Observations and Quantum Electrodynamic calculations by Schulte et al, published as recently as 1998, estimate the size of water clusters as being 280 molecules/cluster at 0°C, and even a non-negligible 3 molecules/cluster at 100°C. In the normal temperature range of biological systems of 30°C–40°C, they found 70–40 molecules/cluster, respectively. [Schulte and Endler, 1998, p. 61]

In 1995, further interesting observations were made by Arani *et al.* [Arani *et al*, 1995] They found coherent regions are not only closely tied with their corresponding electromagnetic field but that they couple strongly with other fields of similar vibration. Such coupling enhances the coherence of the entire structure of water. The actual range of resonant vibrations matches closely the frequencies of many crystals found in nature—which explains why water is such a powerful solvent for many natural substances.

The coupling effect also implies that cluster phenomena are not just local but global—having effects throughout the entire solution. Thus, water prepared in such ways are not merely collections of isolated spherical shells but solution-wide regions of coherence.

Coupling of clusters of similar vibrational frequencies bring to mind the principle of *resonance*. Resonance is a familiar phenomenon, demonstrated well by the tuning fork. Imagine two tuning forks. If one of middle C is struck in the presence of one of F, nothing happens. However, if one of middle C is struck in the presence of one of middle C, the second vibrates as well. Energy is transferred from one to the other depending on similarity of frequency.

The famous story of an opera singer being able to shatter a crystalline goblet with voice alone is another illustration.

Coherent substances have "resonant frequencies" which enable them to couple with others of similar vibration, transferring energy

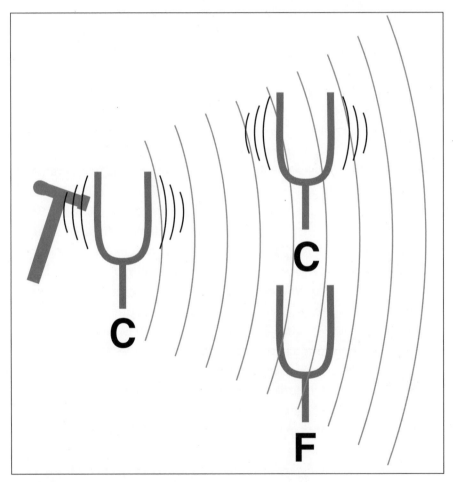

FIGURE 11   Resonance as demonstrated by tuning forks.

and thus information. This concept is central to understanding how homeopathic remedies might work, given the medium of water composed of both random and coherent regions.

Proof of Clusters

The most recent—and significant—research in the physics of coherent water has been done by Dr. S.Y. Lo from the California Institute of Technology and American Technologies Group. [Lo SY, 1996, 1998] He demonstrated, by quantum electrodynamic calculations and actual measurements, the presence of what he calls "I_E™ clusters" of water formed by the process of both serial dilution and shaking. He demonstrated that these clusters are not formed to such a degree by simple dilution without shaking, or mere shaking without diluting.

Dr. Lo's work demonstrates more emphatically than previously the value of adding kinetic energy to the dilution process. Shaking, as is done in homeopathy, is one method. Ultrasound, electrical currents, and other methods suffice as well.

As kinetic energy is applied during dilutional formation of clusters, forces binding clusters together are strengthened, rendering them more stable. Lo finds that I_E water is stable for at least years in duration without significant degradation.

I_E clusters are like microscopic ice in normal water. These clusters are aligned in specific ways which are stable to lengths of 6 molecules to 100 molecules.

Dr. Lo's work is very significant for homeopathy because I_E clusters are prepared by methods very akin to homeopathic potentization. The actual methods used in Dr. Lo's laboratories at American Technologies Group are now secret under proprietary protection, but the solutes are standard salts and even organic molecules, and the process of succussion is improved upon by various modes of imparting kinetic energy. Presumably this represents a more powerful and efficient method of potentizing, which as yet remains to be tested through provings.

Moreover, Dr. Lo has found that the clusters take different structural forms depending on the form of the initiating solute. This corresponds to the Similia quality needed in a remedy.

Dr. Lo's experiments with UV spectroscopy verify that the clusters actually replicate themselves, **even in the absence of the original solute,** because the electromagnetic fields create "meta-stable" states.

Besides proof of both the specificity and ultramolecular nature of Dr. Lo's observations, this research is even more exciting because the measurements are so precise and graphic. A multitude of methods are used to verify the nature and structure of the clusters. It is worth summarizing some of these methods here:

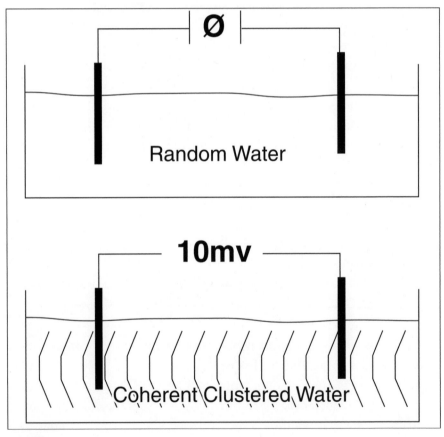

FIGURE 9 Electromagnetic field measurements in normal water and I_E water.

The "electromotive force" of water can be measured by putting two identical stainless steel electrodes in water and measuring the potential. In normal water, there is no potential at all. In I_E water, a finite electromotive force is measured at about 10 mV briefly until thermal activity breaks it down. [Lo SY, 1996]

Transmission electron microscopy has been used to photograph I_E clusters directly. A very dilute solution is filtered through a tiny

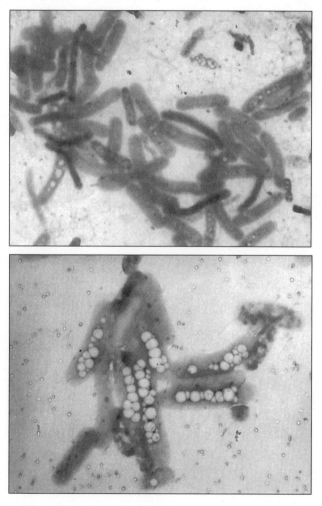

FIGURE 10 Transmission Electron Microscopy photographs demonstrating water clusters of Quantum Electrodynamically predicted sizes.

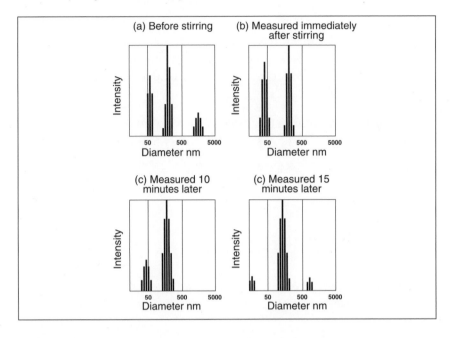

FIGURE 12

Photon Autocorrelation generated by helium-neon laser, showing changes after stirring and then degrading with time. These peaks do not occur in normal or merely shaken water.

filter, then sputter coated with carbon. The carbon coated filter paper is dissolved in boiling chloroform for 20 minutes. Water and I_E structures are dissolved away and only carbon skeletons remain. These are then viewed by an electron microscope. With standard water controls, no structures are seen, whereas I_E clusters show up as linear strings. [Lo SY, 1996] Interestingly, the shape and length of clusters closely match predictions calculated by Quantum Electrodynamics.

With normal water, fluorescence spectrophotometry shows no fluorescence after ultraviolet excitation. With I_E water, however, there are three distinct peaks seen. Dr. Lo's interpretation is that "with a big cluster of molecules in I_E structures, electrons may be shared among different molecules in the same I_E structures, which can be excited by UV light to a new state. Fluorescence light is emitted when the new excited state jumps back to ground state. [Lo SY, 1996] This characteristic demonstrates forces which provide stability to clusters.

Photon Autocorrelation utilizes self-interference of photons generated by a helium-neon laser and enables estimation of the size of I_E clusters. The following figure demonstrates the peaks as they change after stirring. Such absorption is **not** found in **normal** random water used as controls, **nor** in water **merely shaken** with dilution of an initial solute.

Nuclear magnetic resonance (NMR) is a common technique used to measure shifts in the rather fluidly mobile electron cloud/proton arrangement. When a solution is treated with ultrasound, a shift in the NMR peak is unique to I_E clusters and not found in normal, random water. [Lo SY, 1996]

An ingenious method of visibly portraying clusters is Tapping-Mode AFM, which actually traces the height of clusters layered on a mica surface. When correlated with ordinary water, which shows no peaks, and impurities which produce much larger bumps, the pattern of clusters is graphic and convincing.

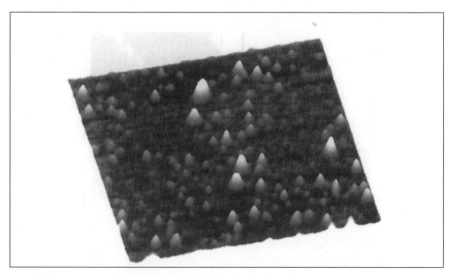

FIGURE 13 Tapping mode AFM, which measures clusters layered on a surface by highly delicate device moving over the surface and raising microscopically.

To me, the most striking and beautiful demonstration of the electrical nature of I_E structures is demonstrated by evaporating monosodium phosphate I_E solutions in the presence of an electromagnetic field. **The resulting pictures can be seen on the back cover of this book.** With ordinary (control) water, monosodium phosphate crystallizes amorphously in the field because the molecules are arranged randomly. With I_E monosodium phosphate solution, the crystals align themselves remarkably with the electromagnetic field in fan-like fashion extending over the full area of the evaporation surface. The result is not only arrayed spatially, but the clusters refract light into striking colors as well. Without using fancy technique, this method shows elegantly and simply how different I_E water is from normal water.

All of the above impressively display the presence and properties of I_E water. Characteristically, it has both specificity of structure and the ability to perpetuate itself. In this sense, the clusters themselves are the active principle. Avogadro's number becomes irrelevant because water is no longer random in such preparations. If water is structured, the presence of the original solute becomes insignificant.

Dr. Lo and others have made a few more observations about I_E water. Dr. Lo found that the electrodes in the electromotive force experiments were very difficult to clean. Somehow, the clusters adhere strongly to surfaces. [Lo SY, 1998] Others discovered that pipes that normally clog up with calcium carbonate sludge clear out swiftly when I_E water is run through them. [Lo SY, 1998] I_E water enhances cracking of petroleum, enhances enzymatic reactions, aids in some household cleaner actions, etc. [Chan KYG *et al*, 1998] Most significantly perhaps is its application in vastly improving the efficiency of automobile catalytic converters, thus potentially reducing pollution in the environment. Many of these are the basis of the formation of a new public company named American Technologies Group.

So far, I_E clusters have been found in as much as 6% of the water it occupies. It has been found that the clusters can be perpetuated even through two distillation cycles. Apparently, heat to boiling does not necessarily destroy all of them in the presence of significant per-centages of clusters. Some probably adhere to the tubing in the dis-tillers, fall into the final effluent and then clone themselves. [Lo SY, talk at NCH, 1998]

This is of interest to homeopaths because it has been found empirically that remedies do not survive above about 120°. To this extent, there may be a difference between I_E water and homeopathic remedies. Another possibility, however, is that research will lead to improvements in methods used to prepare remedies—perhaps gen-erating higher percentages of clusters and enabling greater heat tolerance.

Adherence of clusters to surfaces brings to mind the "grafting" phenomenon mentioned at the beginning of this chapter. By adher-ing to surfaces and then replicating either in water or possibly to sugar, I_E clustering may explain one of the oldest mysteries in homeopathy.

Summary

Homeopathic remedies have distinct properties known for two cen-turies, but devoid of explanation. Recent biophysical research, based on modern Quantum Electrodynamics and development of advanced techniques of measurement, has demonstrated that water prepared by homeopathic methods has regions of coherence and resonance which are capable of replicating clusters and transmitting informa-tion. Thus, the very molecular and electromagnetic structures of coherent water render the paradox of Avogadro's number irrelevant. Finally, research has discovered a mechanism by which information can be stored in homeopathic remedies for communication with bio-logical systems.

Effects on Cells and Tissues

Coherent water is important to understanding how homeopathic remedies can store information for transmission to living organisms, but is it true that such information is transmissible to living cells and tissues? Water being so fundamental to life, it is not difficult to conceptualize that such effects can occur. Nevertheless, systematic investigation requires proof that the specificity and subtlety of homeopathic information truly can be transmitted effectively to organisms.

Fortunately, a plethora of research in laboratories throughout the world have provided such evidence. Much of this pioneering work has been done in Europe because of funding from the European Union, Europe's informal parliament. Hopefully, this represents a trend that will produce dramatic advances not only for homeopathy but for medicine as a whole.

Living organisms are made of organs, which in turn are composed of tissues, the fundamental components of which are individual cells. Cells vary in structure and function but have basic structures in common. The outer layer is a cell membrane made up of lipids (fats) and proteins. Inside (the "cytoplasm") are micro-tubules which transmit molecules, mitochondria which process those molecules and convert them into available energy for use by the cell. Other components provide a variety of specialized functions. Most cells have nuclei, which carry the nucleic acids found in chromosomes. These nucleic acids carry genetic information in chains of specific coded sequences arranged in long, spiral staircase-like structures (called "helical" structures).

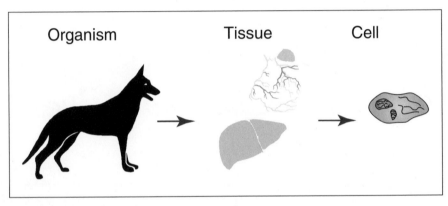

FIGURE 16   Organisms, Tissues, Cells.

At the molecular level, DNA in the nucleus carries the unique genetic codes which characterize each individual and the information needed for individualization of each tissue throughout the body. DNA is copied to a mirrored sequence in RNA which transmits information into the cytoplasm, where proteins called "enzymes" are further copied in specific ways. Enzymes provide a wide variety of functions, but basically they catalyze the complex chemical reactions which drive the cell. Enzymes are true catalysts in that they are not consumed in the process. They merely bring together the molecules into close proximity in order to enable the reactions.

Obviously, the entire process is unbelievably complex in totality. If any portion of the system falters, a cascade of errors can lead to inadequate output of needed functions/products and also a buildup

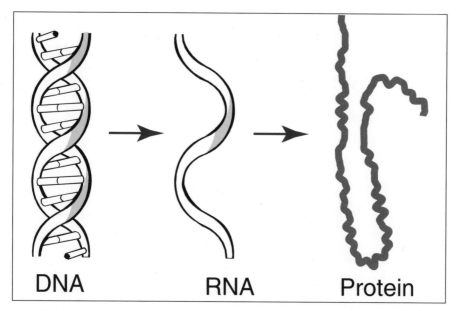

FIGURE 17   DNA to RNA to protein enzyme.

of unneeded molecules—toxic waste products. When running like a finely tuned machine, health results. When disordered, disease occurs.

All of this activity occurs in water, and cannot occur without water. Old concepts of water depended on the idea that molecules were bumping into each other randomly, a basically inefficient mechanism. The beauty of modern concepts of coherent water is that molecules are aligned in orderly fashion, bringing them into contact more directly and efficiently.

Information Theory

It is necessary at this juncture to describe a concept basic to understanding the possible role of remedies in healing: Information Theory. Stated simply, *Water, (and perhaps other polar solvents), can under certain conditions, retain information about substances with which they have previously been in contact, and subsequently transmit this information to presensitized biosystems.* [Fisher P, 1998] Water itself carries information that can be transmitted to living organisms.

But what exactly is "information?"

Biological and chemical systems have traditionally been visualized as a lock/key mechanism. The information is in the structure itself, rather than in the chemical composition of the proteins.

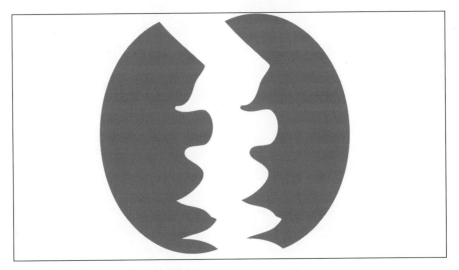

FIGURE 18   A lock and key mechanism.

Or it can be conveyed by sequence, as in a combination lock. This might be the analogy used in DNA to RNA to protein sequence translation. It is known that the genetic material of chromosomes is made of complex strings of helical-shaped strands of DNA. DNA is made up of sequences of units called nucleotides. The sequences are actual codes decoded by enzymes which strip the chains systematically, reading the sequence in a fashion transmitted to create RNA. RNA is known to mirror the code sequence of DNA. RNA code is in turn used to create the structure of proteins which make up the infrastructure and enzymatic functions of all cells.

Enzymes are known to function not only via their sequence of amino acids but also through their three-dimensional structure. The complexity of the amino acid sequence provides electrostatic pressures which help shape the enzyme into a form that optimizes the chemical reaction it is designed to catalyze. In addition, if the pH or chemical environment changes—or if the electromagnetic field changes—the actual three-dimensional form may spring into another shape which catalyzes a different function.

Information transfer can be much more subtle than mere structure would imply. Consider digital communication, such as is seen in computers. A hard disk made of silicon or other metals carry electrical charges, read as on/off or 1/0 switches. Sequences of 1's and 0's convey information. Groupings of these sequences lead to more information, analogous to sentences and paragraphs, folders and files. When transmitted as pixels on screens, the information transforms into graphics and pictures which communicate volumes of information. Send these out over the Internet, and it reaches the entire world. Tell stories in movie form (as in TV) and it evokes whole realms of poetry, drama, spirituality.

Starting from molecular structural switch-like information in 1's and 0's, entire universes of possibilities are conveyed with infinite levels of subtlety and meaning, all of which is real and accessible.

Water appears not only to have measurable structure, but much of the stored information appears to be in the form of electromagnetic fields. The water molecules conform to the fields. Frequencies and vibrations can be measured.

Information transfer implies sending a signal between a transmitter, a transmitting medium, and a sensitive receiver. Like a telephone, radio, or TV system. Resonance, however, is integral to the transmission. Signals which do not resonate with the sensitivity of the receiver are simply not received. That is why we need tuners, channels, or remote controls.

Consider the analogy of two tuning forks. If one has a frequency of C, and the other frequency F, striking the first one has no effect on the second. If, on the other hand, the second also has frequency C, striking the first will cause the second to vibrate also. Further, if

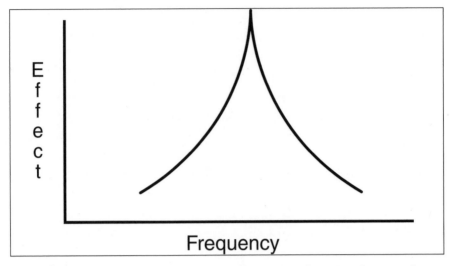

FIGURE 18   Resonance diagram showing peak at "resonant frequency"

the second has a frequency of "C sharp"—not exact but close—the second tuning fork will vibrate but with less intensity. Diagrammatically, resonance can be depicted as in Figure 18.

Another way to express this relationship is: If energy is increased in the transmitter, it will be intensified in the receiver in proportion to the degree of resonance between the two. Upon reflection, it should be easy to see the analogy with potentization and the Law of Similars.

Another example of information transfer, of an analog nature, is music. Consider a Beethoven symphony. A single note communicates one piece of information, but the richness of tone imparts different feelings coming from different instruments in the orchestra. The harmonies and chords plus the lyrics and rhythms add more dimensions. Ultimately, the subtleties can enable one to identify one symphony from another, one composer to another, even one orchestra from another. Each has its own **personality**.

If one symphony creates an inspired feeling, will a second create twice as much inspiration if played together at the same time? Of course not. Dissonance is disturbing and weakens the desired effect.

So transmission of information needs to be done with great accuracy and care in order to be effective. By this analogy, the science of homeopathy also becomes an art of great subtlety. [More on this in Chapter 6]

Therefore, efficiency of cell function still requires that the coherent alignments themselves are correct. If they are off, disorder occurs. Mae-Wan Ho puts the issue nicely:

> The problem of living organization can be stated as follows:
> *How* is it that an organism consisting of a multiplicity of tissues and cells and astronomical numbers of molecules of many different kinds can develop and function as a whole?
> *How* does the organism manage to have energy at will, whenever and wherever required, and in a perfectly coordinated way?"
> [Ho MW, 1998]

The answer lies in the idea that cells, tissues, and indeed whole organisms are themselves **coherent.** Dr. Ho *et al* have provided a technique whereby all levels—from whole organisms to organs to tissues to cells and even to molecules—can be viewed. Based on similar techniques as used in studying crystals in nature, striking and detailed colors are produced by splitting up polarized light into slow and fast rays, passing them through tissues, and then recombining them. The light is refracted by the tissues, causing interference patterns on the output side. The result is patterns of colors which can be finely tuned. [Ho MW, 1993, 1995]

If the molecules in such tissues were randomly organized, the output would be nondescript. Tissues and molecules that are coherent produce distinct colors.

In Dr. Ho's experiments—done on *Drosophila* (fruit fly) larvae—the colors occur coherently throughout the whole organism because the various component vibrations are coupled to each other. This happens even though muscles are moving, energy is transforming, fluids are circulating. Dr. Ho writes, "The *Drosophila* larva—like all other organisms we have looked at, from protozoa to vertebrates without exception—is polarized along the anteroposterior axis, as though the entire organism is one single uniaxial crystal. This leaves us in little doubt that the organism is a singular whole, despite the diverse multiplicity of its constituent parts." [Ho MW, 1998, p. 70]

To carry these observations a step further, Ho found that brief exposures of fruit fly embryos to weak electromagnetic fields cause characteristic global perturbations of their patterns emerging as much as 24 hours later.

Moreover, the perturbations were in phase amongst all the organisms exposed. In order to build up such a phase correlation, the individual fruit flies must phase-lock, or couple coherently, with the others in the population.[Zhou *et al*, 1994]

To re-emphasize a point, recall that such coupled coherence phenomena depend on **resonance** between the organisms.

Dr. Ho's work elegantly demonstrates that cells, tissues, and organisms function in a milieu of electromagnetic coherence. The old biophysics viewed interaction on purely molecular levels. New trends focus on interactions between molecules and electromagnetic fields , as well as between fields themselves.

Related research has been done by Fritz Popp, considered one of the pioneers in detecting ultraweak photon (light) emissions from living systems. He found that these emissions are strongly correlated with the cell cycle and other biochemical functions. [Popp FA, 1992] He later quantified the emissions as being of equal intensity over a broad range of frequencies (200nm to 900nm, which is near the optical range). [Popp FA 1986]

A review of literature by Ho and Popp documents that practically all organisms emit light—some rarely, others very frequently. It is thought that such emissions enable communication between organisms at long distances, a mechanism useful to fish and other marine organisms for the purposes of recognition and defense in the dark. [Ho and Popp, 1994]

As such, communication between organisms is complex. Signals are being passed all the time in realms outside of chemical reactions alone.

Enzymes and Cells in Electromagnetic Fields

Beginning at the most basic level, we review some of the literature demonstrating effects of electromagnetic fields on molecular receptors and enzymes.

In general, protein molecules are capable of rapidly changing from one shape to another depending on their function. These changes occur through complex interactions with other surrounding molecules. Since they are arranged in close proximity, **cooperative interactions occur coherently via mediating electromagnetic fields.** [Frohlich H, 1988; Del Giudice E and Preparata G,1998]

A prime example of such a molecular interaction is rhodopsin, the light receptor in the retina. This is a protein arranged in helical formation attached to a membrane at the base of the retina. When light energy is received (an electromagnetic vibration), the shape of the molecule changes and transfers protons to enhance membrane stability. [Bellavite P and Signorini A, 1998]

Such helical proteins, as glycoproteins called G-proteins, are found in a wide variety of circumstances—such as beta-adrenergic receptors mediating bronchodilation, acetylcholine receptors connecting the nervous system to involuntary muscles, various receptors for neuropeptides in the nervous system, white blood cell receptors enabling recognition of chemicals to be engulfed during inflammations, and recognition systems in yeast cells needed for replication. **These are all receptive to electromagnetic influences.** [Alberts *et al* ,1989]

Parathyroid hormone affects bone cells (osteoblasts) producing bone matrix. This occurs by a receptor which activates an enzyme called adenylate cyclase, and the process is mediated by a G-protein which is inhibited by an electromagnetic field with a 72 Hz frequency and electrical gradient of only 1.3 mV/cm. **This tiny field inhibited the enzyme activity through the G-protein by 90%.** [Adey WR,1988]

A detailed study of the enzyme lysozyme, a prominent participant in inflammatory reactions, shows that its normal inhibition by a competitive inhibitor, n-acetyl glycosamine, can be modulated by weak electromagnetic fields.

> In these experiments, various electromagnetic frequencies were supplied by an oscillator connected to a coil surrounding the test solution. Various frequencies were applied. Interestingly, specific frequencies (40 MHz) increased the effect of the inhibitor, and other frequencies (100 MHz) decreased the effect. Other frequencies (150 MHz) had no effect. Throughout the whole range used, peaks of stimulation and inhibition alternated with no apparent regularity. Closer focus on details between 30 MHz and 50 MHz appeared to show **fractal behavior, which are seen in complex systems in which general patterns are also reflected in finer tuned patterns.** [Shaya SY and Smith CW,1977]

Cyclic adenosine monophosphatase (cAMP) is an important element in controlling the function of many enzymes through transfer of energy. Carefully controlled experimental conditions were set up to measure the activity of cAMP-dependent protein kinases from human lymphocytes. **Electromagnetic waves in a wide range of frequencies inhibited the reaction.**

Type C protein kinase, also cAMP dependent, is important in various cell processes including creation of cancers. This activity was also **modulated by electromagnetic waves.** [Adey WR, 1988]

One of the most interesting pieces of research in this area from a homeopathic perspective is one demonstrating extreme specificity of action at the electromagnetic level. It is generally known that cells have a pumping mechanism to keep sodium (Na^+) ions separated from potassium (K^+) ions. This is moderated by a Na^+/K^+-dependent ATPase enzyme. **A weak electromagnetic field (20 V/cm) is capable of activating the function of this enzyme only if specific**

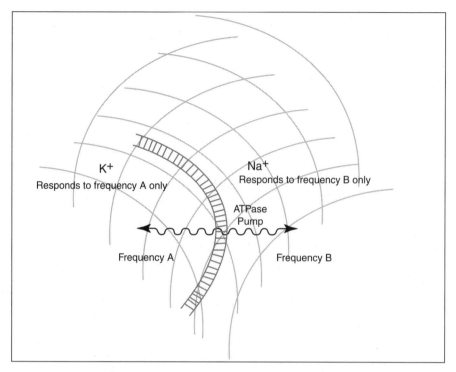

FIGURE 18   Activation of Na/K-dependent ATPase enzyme functioning only if both components are activated by separate resonant frequencies.

frequencies are used simultaneously, each corresponding to opposite sides of the function. Thus, the modulation is dependent on "electroconformational coupling" of a specific resonance. [Tsong TY, 1989]

Finally, DNA itself can be influenced by electromagnetic field interaction. Chromosomal DNA of an insect (larvae of *Acricotopus lucidus*) can be easily viewed under a microscope. It has long been known that when DNA is being transcribed to RNA, the chromosomes uncoil and form puffs. **This process is strongly inhibited** (causing smaller puffs) **by exposure to frequencies of 40-80 GHz and outputs of only 6 mW/cm^2.** The authors noted that the very structure of DNA makes them good candidates for "resonating events." [Kremer F *et al*, 1988]

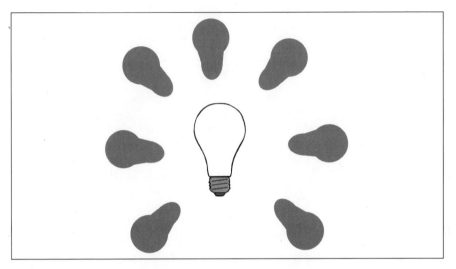

FIGURE 19   Fibroblasts extending filopods in direction of light source.

The next level of complexity occurs in the realm of cells.

Nerve cells in culture and in tissue grow by extending a cone out of one side of the cell, formed by many small protein filaments, called "filopods." **The direction and rate of growth is powerfully influenced by electromagnetic fields, as low as 70 mV/cm.** [Alberts B *et al*, 1989]

Connective tissue cells, called fibroblasts, behave similarly. **3T3 fibroblasts in culture extend filopods preferentially toward light sources,** the most effective being the intermittent ones in the 800–900 nm range with 30–60 impulses per minute. [Albrecht-Buehler G, 1991]

In the previous chapter, Dr. Lo's experiments on I_E water are described in detail. A further outgrowth of this work was research done at UCLA and reported as recently as 1997. A standard system of cultured lymphocytes and monocytes, is used routinely for measurement of various cytokines, intracellular hormones involved in immune inflammatory responses. Measured were activities of tumor necrosis factor alpha (which kills cancer cells), and interleukin-6, interleukin-10, interleukin-12, and interferon-gamma (all of which are involved in protecting cell membranes against viral invasion).

Water Preparation	Cytokine (pg/ml)		
	TNF-a	IL-6	IL-12
Laboratory	260	0	8
ATG Control	260	0	9
I_E#1	12190	3960	1041
I_E#2	10735	4797	1190

FIGURE 20   Cytokine induction by I_E water compared to controls.

Controls were normal laboratory water as well as normal water derived from ATG laboratories (where the I_E water was prepared). Two samples of I_E water, or controls, were added to cell cultures, and the activities of the various cytokines were measured by standardized methods. The outcome was **enhanced activities in the range of thousands-fold over controls.** Once again, the I_E water had nothing in it other than water molecules coherently arranged. Apparently, coherence of the water enhanced the efficiency of cytokine production in the cultured cells. [Bonavida B and Gan XH, 1997]

Effects of Remedies on Cells and Tissues

Electromagnetic field effects are interesting, and perhaps represent the future of medicine in many ways. The question remains, however: What proof is there that homeopathic remedies themselves have similar effects on enzymes, cells, and tissues? Actually, this has been a very dynamic field of research, especially in Europe—and most particularly in recent years. The results are increasingly fascinating as well as convincing. Moreover, as with all pioneering research, even more exciting questions are being raised than answered.

An early study getting attention was done by W. E. Boyd in 1954. A homeopathic preparation was made of *Mercury* and applied to cultures containing an enzyme, malt diastase, responsible for splitting starch molecules. In a meticulous study performed with a very large number of samples over several years, **unequivocal increases in activity were observed despite high dilutions.** [Boyd WE (1954)]

Silver nitrate is known commonly in biology and medicine to stall growth as a normal chemical, yet it is also required as a trace mineral to allow any growth at all.

A study was done in 1926 on the growth of wheat seedlings [Kolisko L,1926], and recently reproduced by four independent researchers including laboratories from the Universities of Graz and of Vienna in Austria. [Lauppert E, 1995] Silver nitrate was prepared by stepwise dilution to 24x (10^{-24}) with 24 agitations between each dilution; this was called D24 by standard European convention. Controls were made by analogously prepared solvent water and by straight unprepared water. Once the D24 baseline of seedling growth was established, a further dilution with agitation was made to D25, which **significantly** *diminished* **the effect** of the test dilution. Most interestingly, **two steps to D26 again** *enhanced* **seedling growth.** This research is significant in the fact that the dilutions exceed Avogadro's number.

This "double switch" kinetic is an observation made frequently in research into remedies at various dilutions. It is verified in practice by homeopaths as well that remedies act optimally at potencies of 6c, 12c, 30c, 200c, 1M, 10M, 50M, and CM. Though somewhat controversial, homeopaths have generally found that intermediate potencies act less well.

Tumor cells have been studied under the influence of various homeopathic compounds which either inhibit or enhance growth. [Bonavida B 1992, 1993]

For a very long time, aspirin has been known to inhibit platelet activity. Platelets are responsible for adherence of blood clots to vessel walls and connective tissue. In recent years, it has been advocated as an effective means to reduce heart attacks. Between 1987 and 1994, **potentized acetylsalicylic acid (aspirin) was also found to reduce bleeding time** due to its action on platelets. [Doutremepuich C *et al*, 1987, 1990, 1994]

This work suggests that the real effect of aspirin on platelets has to do with the electromagnetic field specifically altered by potentized aspirin.

Phytolacca (Pokeroot) has been used empirically by homeopaths for a very long time for mastitis, adenopathy and mononucleosis. *Phytolacca* contains a glycoprotein which is known to induce the transformation of B lymphocytes in culture, which means stimulating the cells to undergo "mitosis" in the process of cell division. B lymphocytes are essential to tissue immunity and are prevalent in the lymphatic system.

In resting lymphocytes, 5c, 7c, and 15c potencies of *Phytolacca* have no mitogenic effect. There is a standard stimulus known as phytohemaglutinin (PHA) which stimulates mitosis. **When the 5c, 7c, and 15c potencies are used in the presence of PHA, they cause a 28–73% inhibitory effect on mitosis.** The maximum effect was found at 15c. [Colas H *et al*, 1975]The same effect was produced at another laboratory in an earlier study, except that the maximum was reached at 7c. [Bildet J *et al*, 1981]

One of the most relevant tissue culture studies in recent years has to do with recovery of rat hepatoma cells from heat damage and/or chemical damage by toxins (sodium arsenite and cadmium chloride). At the cellular level, natural mechanisms of defense and recovery depend on production of so-called "protector proteins."

The results of these studies are very complex but quite interesting:

> First of all, heat shock rendered heightened sensitivity to low dose heat exposure and production of "protector proteins." This can be altered by pretreatments with milder heat. This can be analogous to *isopathic* treatment.
>
> When **sodium arsenite in high dilutions (100 to 300 x 10^{-6})** were applied prior to toxic doses of sodium arsenite, **increased "protector proteins"** were measured in response. This also is an illustration of isopathic treatment.
>
> The Principle of Similars was approximated by pre-treating

cultures with **potentized cadmium chloride.** The cells were **then exposed to cadmium** itself. The idea is that the salt of cadmium is not identical but similar. Instead of having no effect, it **strikingly induced production of "protector proteins."** [Wiegant FAC *et al*, 1993, 1997a, 1997b, 1998]

Similar results have been found in vegetable cells. **Pretreatment with homeopathic dilutions of toxic substances (copper sulphate) protect vegetable cells against the intoxication.** [Guillemain J *et al* 1984, 1987]

It is generally well known that cadmium, an environmental pollutant, and cisplatin, a chemotherapy drug used in cancer treatment, have marked effects on kidney tubules. Very low doses—"high" potencies—of $(10^{-16}M)$ **of cadmium and cisplatin have a protective effect against poisonous doses of each.** [Delbancut A *et al* ,1993]

Research at Montpelier University has studied the effect of epidermal growth factor (EGF) on the proliferation of cultured human keratinocytes and fibroblasts (skin cells). The hormone in very **high dilutions $(10^{-19}M)$ and ultrahigh dilutions $(10^{-45}M)$ caused significant effects.**

Of great interest (other than the observations above Avogadro's number) is that effects were different on each cell type. **Growth was reduced in keratinocytes and stimulated in the fibroblasts.** [Fougeray S *et al* 1993] Thus, the same substance, via the means of electromagnetic effects can have differential effects on cells depending on their resonance and receptivity. Again a demonstration of resonance and the Principle of Similars.

There are two primary types of white blood cells in the immune system. Put simply, lymphocytes produce antibodies, and leukocytes kill by "phagocytosis" (engulfing and digesting foreign substances). These activities are measured by standardized techniques in the laboratory.

Vegetable extracts have long been used in homeopathic doses to produce anti-tumor effects. Wagner's group has studied their component naphthoquinones (plumbagin, alkannin, and others) plus chemotherapeutic agents (vincristine, methotrexate, fluorouracil) at **low dilutions inhibit these immune functions, whereas high dilutions stimulate lymphoblastic transformation and leukocyte phagocytosis.** The dose-response effect is typical. [Wagner H, 1985, 1988a, 1988b, Wagner H, Kreher B, 1989]

A similar complex system was used by Olinescu in Bucharest [Chirila *et al* 1990a and b]. Lymphocytes were stimulated into mitosis by phytohemagglutinin (PHA), granulocytes were stimulated with opsonized zymosan (OZ). Both of these are very standard techniques used in laboratories all over the world.

The cells were isolated from blood drawn from patients either allergic to bee venom or immunodepressed (cancer) patients. Before being stimulated, the lymphocytes were incubated with various dilutions of bee venom, and the granulocytes with various homeopathic

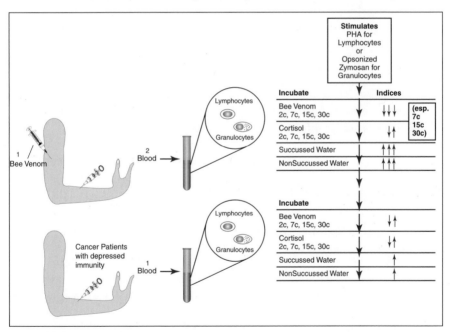

FIGURE 20 Olinescu's Protocol, testing previous cells previously sensitized or depressed, incubating with remedies, and then stimulating artificially. Results demonstrate strong inhibitory effects by potencies of bee venom, and less striking results with phyagocytosis as well as in immunodepressed cancer patients.

dilutions of cortisol (2c, 7c, 14c, 30c). Both in concentrated doses would be expected to have inhibitory effects on the immune indices. As controls, a number of cells were supplemented with succussed or nonsuccussed distilled water.

The lymphocytes of allergic patients were inhibited by the high dilutions of the venom (7c, 15c, 30c). The inhibition did not happen with the controls. the immunodepressed patients had low indices both in the presence and in the absence of venom potencies. **The phagocytosis results were less significant and sometimes contradictory.** It is interesting to note that the different inhibitors behaved differently, although not surprising considering the complexity of the system.

Another approach involved human neutrophils (same as granulocytes) in culture, activated into phagocytosis with formylated peptides which stimulate phagocytes. [Bellavite P *et al,* 1991b, Chirumbolo S *et al,* 1993] They analyzed an extensive series of compounds and several potencies. Results summarized as follows:

> *Manganum phosphoricum* 6x and 8x (manganese phosphate), *Magnesia phosphorica* 6x and 8x (magnesium phosphate), *Acidum citricum* (citric acid), and *Acidum succinicum* 3x and 4x (succinic acid)—**all had significant and reproducible inhibitory effects on the neutrophil's oxidative metabolism.**
>
> *Acidum fumaricum* (fumaric acid) and *Acidum malicum* (malic acid), both at 4x dilution, **had slightly potentiating effects**.
>
> *Phosphorus* and *Magnesia phosphorica* **often presented inhibitory effects,** in the course of various experiments, even at very high dilutions (greater than 15x). These effects occurred but did not always appear at the same dilution, thus nullifying statistical analyses.

These results are relatively soft and hard to interpret meaningfully but nevertheless suggestive. The idea is that similar substances act similarly but differently.

Basophiles are white blood cells primarily found in tissues rather than blood. Under the optical microscope, they are clearly visible and contain colorful granules which can be easily counted. The granules contain histamine, which is central to many allergic phenomena including nasal itching, sneezing, wheezing, and hives. If the basophiles are exposed to IgE antibodies circulating in serum, they are induced to release the histamine. The number of basophilic granules consequently reduce in number and can be quantitatively measured with great precision. This process is called *basophilic degranulation* and is used as a standardized test in immunology laboratories to study the allergic response, the inhibitors/stimulators that affect it, and the drugs that interact with it.

Basophiles are grown easily in tissue cultures and the number of granules are counted easily by standard optical microscopes. Jacques Benveniste in France is one of the pioneering leaders in the use of this technique in immunology in general, and regarding homeopathic potencies in specific. Actually, his team has demonstrated that the degranulation phenomenon is the result of membrane transport rather than to actual direct degranulation. [Beauvais F *et al*, 1991]

The first publications involving the effect of high potencies of homeopathic remedies on basophilic degranulation were done by Poitevan *et al*. It was already known that various allergens (such as house dust mites) caused degranulation. Homeopathic potencies of a remedy known to act powerfully in allergic reactions, *Apis mellifica, or ground honey bee* **(in 9c and 15c), showed inhibition of the degranulation in culture.** [Poitevan B *et al*, 1986]

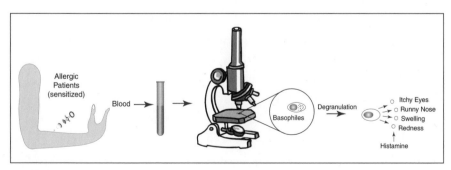

FIGURE 21   Basophilic degranulation method of measuring immune response.

In a further refinement, the basophils were stimulated by **anti-IgE serum, which degranulated them as effectively as the allergens did directly.** The cultures were then exposed to high potencies of *Apis mellifica* and *Lung histamine.* These remedies yielded **significant inhibition at concentrations of 10^{-9} and $^{-17}$ M (9c and 17c).** [Poitevan B *et al,* 1988]

Here the point needs to be made that these remedies are not merely *isopathic*—identical to the allergen. Rather they were truly *homeopathic*—*similar* to the allergen in reaction by the organism.

A further refinement illustrates another point long observed clinically by homeopaths—that there are optimal potencies for clinical effect, which are interspersed on the dilution scale by less effective potencies. This *pseudosinusoidal* dose-response curve was seen in basophilic degranulation experiments as well. **Inhibition was obtained with high dilutions of pure histamine, with inhibition peaks around 6–7c and 17–18c.** [Poitevan B *et al,* 1988, 1990]

A very famous (if not infamous) study was performed under the guidance of Jacques Benveniste in collaboration with four other laboratories. Human basophils were found to be sensitive to infinitesimal doses of substances already known to have stimulatory effects at concentrated doses. These included anti-IgE antibodies, calcium ionophores, and phospholipase A2 (an enzyme).

The controls in this experiment were impressive indeed. It was shown, for example, that the basophils were unresponsive to ultrahigh dilutions of anti-IgG antibodies. It is known that basophils are unresponsive to IgG antibodies in concentrated doses, and this specificity remains at ultrahigh dilutions. Similarly, phospholipase C, which has a different action on membranes than phospholipase A2, shows no effect at ultrahigh dilutions.

Thus, dilution and succussion alone are not significant. Rather, a degree of specificity that matches the homeopathic Principle of Similars holds true. [Davenas E *et al,* 1988]

The dose-response curves in this experiment corroborated those seen previously.

The dose-response curves showed that decreasing doses were accompanied first by disappearance of activity, then by its reappearance and then by various alternating activity peaks and inactivity troughs up to very high dilutions, corresponding to practically zero antibody concentrations. [Davenas E *et al,* 1987]

The effect of succussion was measured by comparison with controls as well. Succussion in Benveniste's laboratories is done by a standard "vortex" such as is used in clinical laboratories to mix blood or serum samples.

It is also reported that in order to obtain maximum activity at the infinitesimal dilutions the dilution process needed to be accompanied by vigorous succussion (10 sec. with a vortex)... [Davenas E *et al,* 1987]

Finally, the most provocative of all of the observations in these pioneering studies:

... the stimulatory activity of the diluted antibody solutions persisted even after ultrafiltration through membranes with a pore size of less than 10 kDa, which should have retained the antibody out of solution. [Davenas E *et al,* 1987]

Thus, the possibility of the degranulation being caused by proteins, however dilute, is ruled out. Yet the effect itself remained!

These studies were published in the well-known journal *Nature,* and were followed by some embarrassing editorial responses. The observations that such high dilutions could have such effects were derided as being in complete violation of the existing paradigms in medicine. Outrageously, a team of investigators led by a magician were sent to debunk the results! Rather than challenge the results directly via scientific means, a sensationalistic and prejudiced report was hurriedly generated to produce an appearance of editorial balance and responsibility. Nevertheless, the paper was published and the results have remained open to reproduction in other laboratories.

The next stage beyond cell culture observations is experimentation upon isolated organ tissues under controlled laboratory conditions.

Such systems have been standardized to degrees of general acceptance in the scientific community for purposes not solely restricted to homeopathy. Thus, any effects created by homeopathic remedies must stand on their own rather than as procedural aberrations.

One such model is isolated guinea pig trachea, in which standard research demonstrates relaxation of tracheobronchial muscle in the presence of beta$_2$-agonists such as isoproterenol, salbutamol, and tulobuterol—components of common asthma inhalers. In a classic demonstration of homeopathic effectiveness, **high dilutions from 10^{-20}M to 10^{-36}M were capable of inducing the same relaxation.** Once again, it needs to be pointed out that Avogadro's number—the point at which no molecule of the original substance no longer exists—is 10^{-24}! [Callens E *et al*, 1993]

Aconitum napellus and *Veratrum album* are known to be toxic to the heart in concentrated form. At low dilutions (high concentrations) of 10^{-5}M, *Aconitum napellus* causes fibrillation in the isolated eel heart perfused by nutrient fluids. At medium dilutions (10^{-7}M), it caused the heart to slow down. And at high dilution, (10^{-18}M), it showed no effect on the heart at all. However, in hearts previously toxified by low dilutions of *Aconitum napellus*, **the high dilutions offered strikingly protective effects at 10^{-18}M.** [Aubin M, 1984, Pennec JP, Aubin M, 1984]

Similar results were obtained with *Veratrum album* on isolated perfused hearts. [Pennec JP *et al*, 1984a, 1984b]

Such research not only confirms isopathic effects on cardiac pathology, but nicely demonstrates the protective effect of high potencies of commonly used remedies.

Jacques Benveniste once again has pioneered immune studies utilizing this model of isolated and perfused guinea pig hearts. The beauty of this system is that it provides a precise measure of cardiac flow, which can be altered by various mixtures of drugs, antagonists, etc. Benveniste has shown that guinea pig heart is also sensitive to immunization-dependent activation. Once immunized with ovalbumin and then isolated between the 9th and 20th day, an increase in

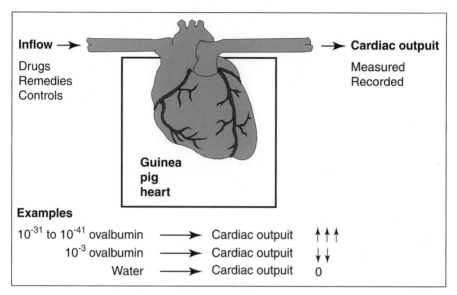

FIGURE 22   Benveniste's standardized guinea pig heart experiments diagrammatically depicted.

coronary flow could be achieved at extremely high dilutions of 10^{-31} to 10^{-41} of ovalbumin. Once again, an isopathic observation, but a powerful demonstration of the effectiveness of substances potentized beyond Avogadro's number. [Benveniste J, 1992; Litime MH *et al*, 1993]

At this point, Benveniste launches into truly revolutionary research.

> Closed ampoules of histamine, ovalbumin or LPS, and water (as controls) were placed inside a coil through which an electric current was passed. An amplifier then delivered the current to another coil in which was inserted a closed ampoule of water. The water treated with the current from the coils with histamine, ovalbumin and LPS and perfused through the guinea-pig heart was **capable of increasing coronary flow. The water treated with the current from the coil containing water, on the other hand, had only a minimal effect. The differences were highly significant (p<0.001).** [Aissa J *et al*, 1993; Benveniste J *et al*, 1994b]

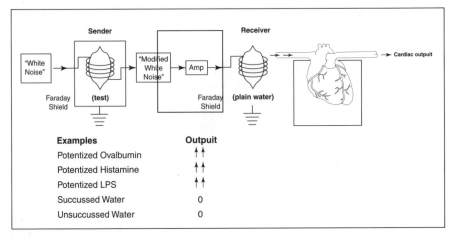

Examples	Outpuit
Potentized Ovalbumin	↑↑
Potentized Histamine	↑↑
Potentized LPS	↑↑
Succussed Water	0
Unsuccussed Water	0

FIGURE 23   My diagrammatic representation of Benveniste's transference of information ampoule to ampoule via amplified electric current, altering water in the second ampoule such that it could stimulate cardiac outflow in guinea pig hearts.

At a recent talk delivered at Stanford Medical School on June 7, 1999, Benveniste reiterated these results and added some refinements. Into a Faraday-cage protected environment, "white noise" was transmitted by an oscilloscopic source through the experimental sample held in a polyethylene test tube. The resulting modulated signal was picked up at the other end and then amplified. When applied in amplified form to another tube with ordinary water, the water was added to the perfused guinea pig heart for measurement of cardiac flow.

When ordinary water is used in the sump, no change in cardiac output occurs.

When diluted and succussed ovalbumin is transmitted oscilloscopically to ordinary water under these conditions, the resulting water increases the cardiac flow, even though only exposed to an electromagnetic field in a near-acoustic range of 10 to 100 Hz! There is no molecule of ovalbumin present!

Finally, the most astounding result reported by Benveniste is that **the modulated "white noise" can be digitized and placed**

on a CD or computer —just as music is recorded for playing on CD or computer. And then, of course, this information is transmissible by the Internet, say from Chicago to France, as demonstrated by Benveniste! And the water exposed after such transmission and amplification still is able to increase cardiac flow!

To the human ear, such sounds sound like a whisper or a whooshing sound. But embedded within these frequencies are specific signals belonging to potentized ovalbumin. In a receptor prepared specifically to receive such signals—pretreated guinea pig heart—the result is measurable. Remember, no molecule is involved in this entire translation except as the original solute for the potentization process. All the rest is in the form of highly specific electromagnetic signals. [Benveniste, June 7,1999, talk delivered at Stanford Medical School]

Summary

Having established coherent water as connected to specificity and resonance to electromagnetic fields, the next step is to demonstrate that such influences affect living organisms. Numerous examples of electromagnetic field effects are seen in enzymes, cell cultures, and isolated organ tissues. Furthermore, homeopathic remedies demonstrate similar phenomena. Most significantly for the future of biophysics in general and homeopathy in particular, recent research shows that highly specific signals can be transmitted electromagnetically, and stored digitally, via the medium of water in highly precise laboratory protocols. These can then be transmitted over great distances in order to reproduce results.

CHAPTER

5

Transmission to Living Organisms

As we have seen, coherent water clusters and electromagnetic interactions—most particularly in the form of homeopathic remedies—have demonstrable effects on simple cells and tissue cultures in laboratories. Proof in the pudding, however, is in whole living organisms in all their complexity.

Coherence itself has already been described in *Drosophila* larvae by Ho et al. [Ho MW *et al* 1993, 1995] To reiterate, larvae were found to coherently refract plane-polarized light as whole organisms—in like manner to crystals—although made of individual components. Without exception, **the light was polarized along anteroposterior axes** of the organism. Moreover, X-ray diffraction reveals that a high degree of supramolecular order is maintained even during isometric muscular contractions. [Bordas J *et al* 1993]

Humans demonstrated coherence as well in a series of classic studies done by Smith *et al* in collaboration with allergologists from hospitals in London and Dallas, Texas. They found that certain human individuals were "sensitive" to minimal perturbations of electromagnetic fields. These hypersensitive patients exhibited a variety of acute allergic symptoms when exposed to the allergens to which they were sensitive. This was expected and predictable.

The striking observation was that the **exact same symptomatology was induced by simply bringing the patients into close contact with sources of electromagnetic radiation**—in particular frequency bands ranging, according to individual patients, from only a few mHz to a large number of MHz. Importantly, it was not so much the intensity of the output (a few V/m) as the " *frequency* and *coherence*" that activated the symptoms. [Smith CW *et al*, 1985; Monro 1987, Smith 1988, Smith 1989,1994]

The next discovery in these experiments was that not only did the hypersensitive patients respond to electromagnetic frequencies, but the **patients themselves produced electromagnetic signals during the allergy attacks.** These signals were produced regardless of whether the attacks were initially induced by electromagnetic radiation or the chemical allergens themselves. Clearly, the process of an allergy attack in such individuals is sensitive to both reception

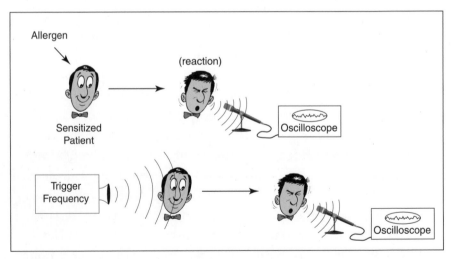

FIGURE 24   Specific allergens given to a sensitized patient trigger an allergic reaction. Specific triggering frequencies in the proximity of the patient can also trigger an attack. In either case, once in an attack, specific frequencies emitted by the patient can be detected and recorded by an oscilloscope.

and emission of electromagnetic radiation—a close interaction between fields and biophysical and inflammatory reactions.

A similar phenomenon is found in several species of fish capable of perceiving and responding to electric field intensities in similar ranges as those in allergic patients (1 µV/m). [Bullock TH, 1997] It is conceivable that fish use these sensitivities to detect food and predators at great distances in the wild.

An extremely fascinating outcome of Smith's research for our purposes was the observation that allergic attacks in the select population of hypersensitive patients could be *neutralized* **by exposure to certain frequencies of radiation.** That is, the patient is first triggered by a chemical agent, and the reaction is then stopped by

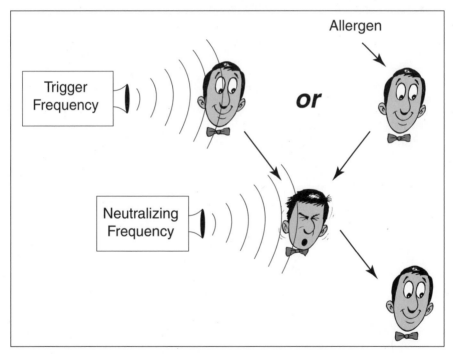

FIGURE 25 Frequencies which resonate with the individual patient can duplicate or neutralize an allergic reaction if matched closed to the hypersensitive individual. Either an allergen or a trigger frequency create a reaction, as in the previous figure. Once a reaction is established, a neutralizing frequency will stop the reaction.

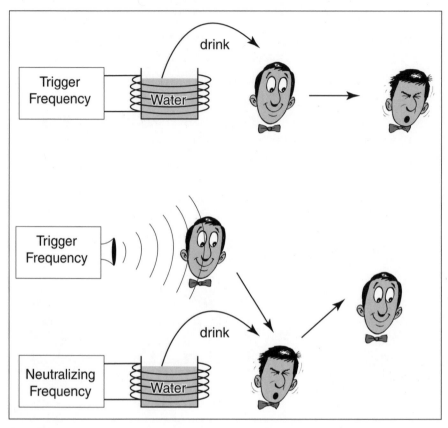

FIGURE 25 Water that has been treated by either specific triggering frequencies or specific neutralizing frequencies will have the corresponding effect when drank by the patient.

appropriate electromagnetic frequencies. Most fascinating of all is the fact that **water itself, after exposure to the appropriate frequency, could also neutralize the attack when drank by the patient.** Furthermore, water exposed to other frequencies known to trigger attacks would trigger an allergic reaction in turn.

Thus, water itself can be a medium of transmission of electromagnetic information to allergic humans of appropriate sensitivity—either neutralizing or triggering attacks by respective and very specific frequencies. This phenomenon comes closest to demonstrating homeopathic influences (or at least isopathic) as possible without using actual remedies.

Solutions can be serially diluted and succussed and then measured by scanning several oscillators in a frequency range of 0.1 Hz to 10 MHz. The subtle "reaction" of each "potency" field was then measured by a test person's microtremor. Thus, **patterns of resonant frequencies over ranges of dilutions have been established.** The control—untreated water—showed a frequency of 8.0 MHz. At other dilutions, **clusters of resonance occurred in alternating biphasic fashion around frequencies of 3, 7, 10, 12, 16, 19, 90 Hz.** [Smith CW *et al*, a collaboration described in Endler PC, Schulte J, 1994]

Clearly, water can be a medium of transmission of highly specific information. Such measurements may be the beginning of a database of "natural" resonant frequencies which can help standardize future research. Such standardization would be valuable for elucidating the mechanism of action of homeopathic remedies. As more is understood about these phenomena, better controls can be created for more sophisticated experiments. In addition, the biphasic phenomenon at different dilutions can be more precisely understood—as to whether it is a classical interference phenomenon, or some other mechanism.

More practically, standardization of this type enables "assay" techniques which can demonstrate the potency of a given remedy— a tremendous boon to homeopathic pharmacies seeking to provide quality control for their products. Correspondingly, practitioners and patients who question whether a given prescription was accurate or whether the remedy was spoiled can test its true quality.

Before proceeding, a few points need to be made about phases in healing, especially in regard to experimental outcomes. When dealing with whole organisms, complex processes are involved. It can be difficult to define a proper endpoint for evaluating the effectiveness of a homeopathic remedy—or any other treatment, for that matter. It is not enough to isolate a featured effect and then equate that with

healing as a whole. Nevertheless, science proceeds by such reductionistic methods. We just need to be cognizant of this limitation as
we continue.

On a theoretical level, P. Bellavite and A. Signorini have described
a useful model for considering phases in healing. [Bellavite P, Signorini A, 1998] Traditionally, diagnostic criteria (say, liver function
or kidney function tests, or EKG disturbances or X-rays) are used
to define sickness. These, however, represent the last stages in a
process.

The first stage is characterized by tiny disorders from custom-
ary functioning. These fluctuations render the organism susceptible
to perturbations induced by external agents of any kind—say, emotional, physical, or even electromagnetic or chemical. This stage is
not quite sickness in itself. Rather, it is a **predisposition** to falling
sick. The borderline here is extremely hazy but nevertheless real.

At this stage, what might be a stress to a predisposed individual would be shrugged off lightly by a healthier person. In addition,
the difference here might not be so much one of quantity of "strength"
as a resonance phenomenon. An otherwise flexible person might
succumb quickly to a particular sensitivity, as in Smith's allergic
subjects.

The second stage occurs when the organism shifts into a reaction in order to establish a kind of homeostasis or balance in the
midst of weakness. Classically this is seen as the **inflammatory** stage
of illness. The immune system is mobilized to expel foreign invaders
or create pain around a joint so as to prevent further motion damage. A variety of reactions come into play here—including neurological, endocrine, psychological, and circulatory. At first, these
processes are necessary to prevent further damage. However, they
concomitantly produce damage in themselves. The organism has
been prevented from experiencing disaster but now is burdened with
the "water damage following fire fighting."

An important point is that this second stage is still somewhat
functional. With proper care and treatment, the organism may be

capable of returning to its original state. This is unlikely to occur, however, with merely minor adjustments in lifestyle, etc. Rest and therapeutic attention are required to shift the equilibrium back to normal.

The third phase of the disease process occurs when the organism fails to cope. Deposition of toxins, excessive proliferation of cells (as in cancer), shifting of receptor sensitivities (as in drug tolerance or pain tolerance), and permanent biochemical and anatomical changes—all may occur in this stage. Here the adaptation itself is having **degenerative** effects which may become semi-permanent. A cascading effect shifts stress from one organ to another.

This description helps the clinician understand the process of disease and its consequences more clearly. Moreover, Bellavite and Signorini point to pioneering thinking which is likely to shape the future of medicine in general:

> From a biophysical standpoint, disease may be regarded not only as a functional or molecular-structural abnormality, as in the classic view, but also (and not by way of contrast) as a disturbance of an entire network of electromagnetic communications based on long-range interactions between elements (molecules, nerve centers, organs, to mention but a few) which oscillate at frequencies which are coherent and specific and thus capable of resonance." [Bellavite P, Signorini A, 1998]

Isopathic Research

Bearing in mind these principles, a plethora of studies have been reported of value to our thesis.

A team of American researchers have reported results of very high dilutions of mice tissues infected with *Francisell tularensis,* a nosode. Homeopathic **nosodes** are pathological products from animals or humans that are then diluted and succussed into potencies. In this case, potentizations were made from reticulo-endothelial tissue (immune tissue) of mice infected with tularemia, a fatal disease. Three dilutions below Avogadro's number (3x, 7x, and 12x) and three dilutions beyond there being any molecule of original substance (30c, 200c, and 1000c) were tested.

These preparations were administered orally to a group of mice, whereas another control group was treated with dilutions of ethanol. Toxic doses of the *F. tularensis* organism were administered. Total mortality of the mice was the endpoint measured.

After 15 experiments, the **high potencies were found to cause a significant increase in survival time and a significant reduction in total mortality compared to controls.** Protection did not correlate with the level of dilution, number of shakings, or presence or absence of original tissue when all potencies were compared. [Jonas WB, *et al*, 1991]

A standard study system in immunology involves mice thymus gland. A hormone from the thymus (thymulin) was administered in potencies of 4c, 7c, 9c, or 11c. When given to healthy mice, **specific blood and cellular immune response measurements were significantly *depressed* with the highest dilutions. When thymulin was given to immunodepressed mice (via genetic or surgical means), the potencies caused a significant *stimulation* of the same measurements.** [Doucet-Jaboeuf M, *et al*, 1982; Bastide M, *et al*, 1985, 1987, 1995]

A well-defined protocol has been devised to study production of cancers in rats in the presence of various carcinogenic substances. To summarize a complex experimental system, a large percentage of rats who were given diets with 2-acetylaminofluorene (0.03% for 21 days) and phenobarbital (0.05% for 12 months) developed liver cell cancers after 9–20 months. These served as controls. Treatment of the animals with 2-acetylaminofluorene 9c or with phenobarbital 9c added to the drinking water **significantly reduced and delayed development of liver tumors in comparison with a control group** given only the solvent water diluted and succussed. [De Gerlache J and Lans M, 1991]

A very interesting study bearing on the physiological action of remedies was done at the Department of Zoology of the University of Santiniketan (India) by Sukul *et al.* Rats were kept on a high-salt diet, anesthetized, and a microelectrode connected to an oscilloscope was implanted in the lateral hypothalamic area of the brain. After a suitable time period recording the baseline tracing of discharge frequencies, a few drops of *Natrum muriaticum* (sodium chloride, table salt) in potencies of 30c and 200c were applied to the tongue. **Marked reductions in the hypothalamic discharge frequencies occurred.** This research demonstrated that one mode of transmission can be by nerve transmission, and that a high-salt diet presensitizes rats to the corresponding isopathic remedy. [Sukul NC, *et al*, 1993]

Isopathic treatment has been researched extensively in the context of detoxification. In a typical protocol, an isopathic potency of a poison is given before or after an animal is poisoned in order to compare survival with that of control groups.

In a series of old studies, plants poisoned by toxic doses of a copper salt were treated with potencies of the same salt. **In all cases, the plants recovered.** [Netien G, *et al*, 1965; Boiron J & Marin J, 1967; Noiret R & Glaude M, 1976; Projetti ML, *et al*, 1985]

In another isopathic study, kidney toxicity in rats pretreated with **9c and 15c dilutions of *Mercurius corrosivus*** (Corrosive sublimate of Mercury) were **significantly protected from death against toxic doses of Mercury** (5–6 mg/kg). This observation has been extensively reproduced in a variety of laboratories. [Cambar J, *et al*, 1983; Guillemain J, *et al*, 1984; LaRue F and Cal JC, 1985; LaRue F, *et al*, 1986; Cal JC, *et al*, 1986, 1988 a, b; LaRue F, *et al*, 1985]

Gentamycin is an antibiotic known to have kidney toxicity. In rats poisoned with Gentamycin, **potentized Gentamycin protects the rat kidneys.** [Souza Magro LA, *et al*, 1986]

Alloxan is known to produce diabetes in mice. *Alloxan* **9c partly inhibits the diabetogenic effect of a dose of 40 mg/kg of Alloxan.** Of significance is the fact that the potency acted both preventively (if given beforehand) and curatively (if given afterward). [Cier A, *et al*, 1966]

Arsenic poisoning of rats has been studied extensively, with recovery after administration of isopathic *Arsenicum album.* [Cazin JC, 1986; Boiron J and Cier A, 1962 a, b, 1971; Boiron J, *et al,* 1968, 1978; Cazin JC, *et al,* 1987; Chaoui A, 1988; Gaborit JL, 1987]

In the most classic study of this genre, rats were treated with toxic doses (10mg/kg) of arsenic trioxide. Homeopathic dilutions were then injected intraperitoneally (into the abdomen for enhanced absorption via the intestines). **Blood levels and urinary excretion were measured** over time thereafter. In a series of dilutions (5c, 7c, 9c, 11, 13, 15, 17, 19c, 21c, 23c, 25c, 27c, 29c, and 31c), the most active dilutions were 7c, 17c. [Cazin JC, *et al,* 1991]

In this experiment, an interesting control was used—water alone diluted and succussed but without the arsenic trioxide. This showed very significant differences from test potencies but no difference from unsuccussed water. Moreover, it is of note that the protective effect of the high dilutions was abolished if they were subjected to heating to 120 degrees for 30 min.

True Homeopathic Studies

Isopathic studies are well and good, but the homeopathic principle relies on the use of *similar* substances.

A number of studies have demonstrated that 7c potencies of arsenic and bismuth are capable of increasing the urinary elimination of these same metals by rats intoxicated by them. Interestingly from the homeopathic viewpoint, **potentized arsenic had no effect on bismuth intoxication and vice versa**. [Lapp C, *et al,* 1955, Wurmser L and Ney J, 1955]

Another combination of isopathy and homeopathy is a study on rats treated with lethal doses of a-amanitine (the poison of the mushroom *Amanita phalloides*). **15c potencies of amanitine, *Phosphorus,* and rifampicin significantly slowed mortality compared to controls.** [Guillemain J, *et al,* 1987]

Phosphorus is known to be hepatotoxic in high doses, and *Phos-*

phorus is frequently used by homeopaths in liver cases when the totality of symptomatology fits. Rifampicin may be similar to amanitine in terms of mechanism of action, which is inhibition of enzymatic activity such as that of RNA polymerase). So, if the mechanism of action is similar, high potencies may be capable of action even in the presence of a lethal dose of poison.

Phosphorus **in 30c potency has been shown to have a protective effect on fibrosis of the liver caused by chronic administration of CCl$_4$** (carbon tetrachloride) to rats. This was further corroborated by a **decrease in serum hepatic enzymes** compared to a group of untreated rats. [Palmerini CA, *et al*, 1993] Once again a verification of the Principle of Similars.

A final but interesting study was performed at the Department of Zoology of the University of Kalyani (India). Albino mice were irradiated with 100–200 rad of X-rays (sublethal doses) and evaluated after 24, 48, and 72 hours. Cell damage was measured by frequency of chromosomal aberrations, formation of micronuclei, and the mitotic index (rate of cell reproduction). Homeopathic *Ginseng* 6x, 30x, and 200x and *Ruta graveolens* 30x and 200x were administered orally before and after irradiation. **the mice treated with the homeopathic remedies suffered less damage to a "spectacular" degree than the control mice** (which were irradiated and treated with doses of ethanol). [Khuda-Bukhsh AR and Banik S, 1991]

Many experiments have been performed measuring so-called "first aid" effects of traditional remedies.

Homeopathic *Silica* is frequently used in wound healing, particularly when suppurations have developed. Its effect was found to be **curative in wound healing in mice.**[Oberbaum M, 1992]

On experimental model from Rehovot (Israel) used the repair of holes pierced in the ears of mice as a measure of the effect of homeopathic *Silica* in dilutions up to 200c, added to drinking water for 4–20 days. The **homeopathic *Silica* healed lesions faster and brought about a greater reduction in their size than sodium chloride solutions used as a control.** [Oberbaum M, *et al*, 1991, 1992]

Another *Silica* study demonstrated its effects of Platelet Activation Factor, which is a step in wound healing—in this case produced by peritoneal macrophages in the mouse. *Silica* was added to drinking water at the 9c dilution for 25 days. The macrophages extracted from the mice thus treated showed a **PAF production** capability upon provocation by yeast extracts which **was 30 to 60% greater than that of control macrophages**—untreated mice, mice treated with NaCl in 9c dilution or with another homeopathic drug, *Gelsemium* (Yellow Jasmine) 9c. Interestingly, in conformity with the biphasic or sinusoidal dose-response seen in other studies, a lower dilution of 5c had no effect. [Davenas E, *et al*, 1987]

One of the most archetypical studies done to illustrate the Similia Principle was the administration of potentized bee venom in albino guinea-pigs on X-ray-induced erythema (redness). These studies have been duplicated in other laboratories without difficulty.

In nature, bee stings cause a similar edema and erythema. *Apis* **7c had a protective effect and roughly 50% curative effect on the X-ray burns.** [Bastide M , *et al*, 1975; Poitevin B, 1988b, Bildet J, *et al*, 1990] This observation correlates nicely with tissue culture studies in which *Apis* inhibits histamine release from basophilic degranulation (Chapter 4).

In a complementary study, the effect of homeopathic remedies on induced edema in the foot of a rat were evaluated. Potencies of histamine up to 30x were injected intraperitoneally into rats before and simultaneously with injection of inflammatory doses of histamine (0.1 mg) into the foot. **A small, but statistically significant inhibitory effect was noted.** [Conforti A, *et al*, 1993]

Homeopathy is used extensively in labor/delivery and postpartum periods in both humans and animals.

In pigs, remedy combinations have both **prophylactic and therapeutic effects on infections (metritis and mastitis) of sows and on diarrhea of piglets.** The combinations used were: *Lachesis* (venom of the bushmaster snake), *Pulsatilla* (Windflower), and *Sabina* (savin) or *Lachesis, Echinacea* (Coneflower), *Pyrogenium* (nosode made from sepsis), and *Caulophyllum* (Blue Cohosh). The potencies used ranged from 1x to 6x. [Both, 1987]

A related effect on a variety of postpartum complications of dairy cows was demonstrated by *Sepia* (ink of the cuttlefish) 200c. [Williamson AV, *et al*, 1991]

Cuprum (copper) has long been used in homeopathy when the totality of symptoms characteristically involves a prominence of spasms or cramps. A French team [Santini R, *et al*, 1990] developed an animal model for assessing the possible effect of *Cuprum* on digestive motility. A 4c potency was administered intraperitoneally to mice, which then received neostigmine in doses of 50 mg/kg—a drug which normally accelerates intestinal motility. The parameter measured was the distance travelled by phenolsulphonphthalein die in the intestine. *Cuprum* **4c significantly reduced transit time** in rats treated with neostigmine, returning them back to transit times closer to control rats that were not treated at all with neostigmine. Copper itself, administered alone, had no effect.

Chelidonium is a homeopathic remedy known to have profound effects on liver and gallbladder cases when given as part of a total picture of symptoms. One study demonstrated that *Chelidonium* 3c was able **to cure rats with induced hypercholesteremia.** [Baumans V, *et al* ,1987]

Complex research on immunostimulatory effects of remedies in mice was conducted extensively by Bastide and co-workers. There are two major types of immunity: humoral (or blood circulated) and cellular (or tissue-bound). Humoral measurements of immune function is done by counting the number of plaque-forming cells produced when the organism is stimulated. Cellular immunity is measured by T-cell killer cells in response to immune stimuli specific for those particular cells. These are standardized parameters used throughout the scientific community.

A wide variety of experiments were made by Bastide's group [Doucet-Jaboeuf M, *et al*, 1982, 1984 Bastide M, 1985; Doucet-Jaboeuf M, *et al*, 1985 Bastide M, *et al*, 1987; Guillemain J, *et al*,

1987; Daurat V, *et al,* 1988] Among the results were those describing thee effects of high dilutions (in the range corresponding to 5c) of α-b interferon (a viral protective agent) and thymic hormones (immune system hormones). **The remedies had definitive stimulatory effects on immune function.** The authors even suggested that they might be useful for treatment in immunodepressed patients. [Bastide M, *et al,* 1985]

Another complex set of experiments were conducted by Bentwich and coworkers. [Weisman Z, *et al,* 1992a, 1992b] Previously, an antigen called KLH (hemocyanin) in 6c and 7c potency were capable of specifically modulating antibody response in experimental animals. [Toper R, *et al,* 1990] They repeated and expanded on these experiments by focussing on mice. The mice were preconditioned for 8 weeks with intraperitoneal injections of potencies of KLH antigen 7c and 8c, as well as saline as a control. They were then immunized with KLH in a routine manner. Serum levels of specific antibodies were determined by immunoassay. **The results showed a significant increase in specific IgM antibody response with all the preconditioning dilutions.** In addition, there was **a significant increase in specific IgG response in animals pretreated by KLH 18c,** which is far beyond Avogadro's number. The authors conclude that it is possible to stimulate immunity with dilutions even beyond Avogadro's number.

Complex and Convincing Homeopathic Studies

One of the most elegant demonstrations of the Principle of Similars, in my opinion, was performed on a system in which salivary glands are stimulated to expand in size within 14 days and then return to normal within another 30 days. It is known that two substances reliably produce this response: isoproterenol (commonly found in asthma inhalers) and eleidosin (an intracellular hormone). Both have the same effect.

In the experiment, isoproterenol was administered in material doses as usual to the rats, while eleidosin was given in dilutions ranging from 10^{-10} to $^{-426}$ g/ml. The **response was significant compared to controls,** both in terms of preventing the increase in size of the glands and in accelerating their return to normal size. Thus, compounds having similar action can interact in homeopathic potency even beyond Avogadro's number. [De Caro G, *et al,* 1990]

Another "pure" demonstration of the Similia Principle demonstrates that immunity can be stimulated by ultrahigh dilutions in absent immune systems. It is known that B lymphocyte production is dependent upon the "bursa of Fabricius" in chickens. In this study, bursectomy was performed in chick embryos, rendering them severely immunodeficient.

The hormone bursin in dilutions ranging up to 10^{-30} to $^{-40}$g/ml—far beyond Avogadro's number—were injected into the eggs. **A normal adult antibody response occurred upon later stimulation with the antigen bovine thyroglobulin.** Controls, of course, showed no antibody response whatsoever by contrast. Moreover, **a normal pituitary-adreno-cortical axis was shown by measurement of adrenocorticotropic hormone,** which was impossible in the controls. [Youbicier-Simo BJ, *et al,* 1993; Bastide M, 1994]

Landmark Study in Tadpoles

A 1998 report by Endler *et al.* ties together most of the principles presented in the research thus far. This research is important because it utilizes well-established standardized procedures, and the experiments have been duplicated by ten individual researchers at eight different European university centers.[Endler J and Schulte J, 1998]

Tadpoles from grass tree frogs were studied in their development. It had been noted previously that **thyroxin up to a dilution of 10^{-8} induces and accelerates metamorphosis** from larvae to tadpoles. The endpoint can be measured precisely by the point at which the feet break out of their enclosing membrane. **Homeopathically prepared (dilution/succussion) solutions of 10^{-11} to 10^{-30} actually inhibit** the metamorphosis of the larvae. Control water

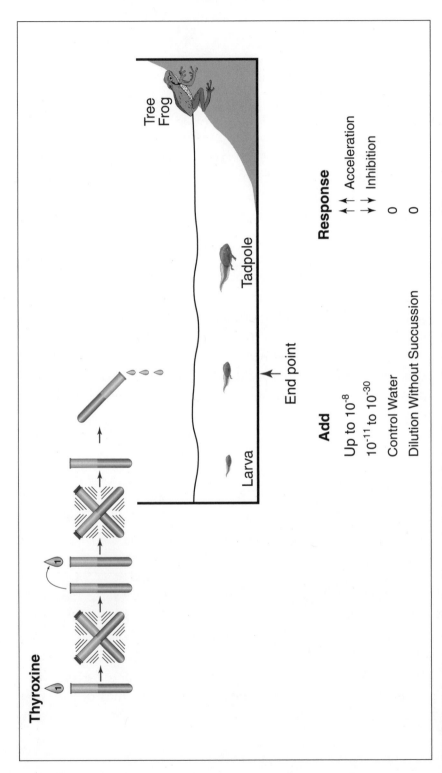

FIGURE 27 Metamorphosis of larvae to tadpoles to tree frogs as affected by various potencies of thyroxine

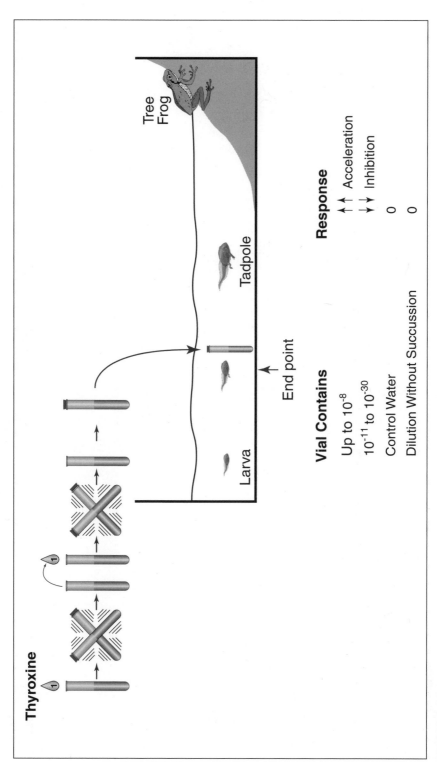

Thyroxine

Vial Contains

Up to 10^{-8}

10^{-11} to 10^{-30}

Control Water

Dilution Without Succussion

Response

← ← Acceleration

→ → Inhibition

0

0

FIGURE 28 Metamorphosis altered by potentized thyroxine inside a *sealed glass vial* placed in basin water.

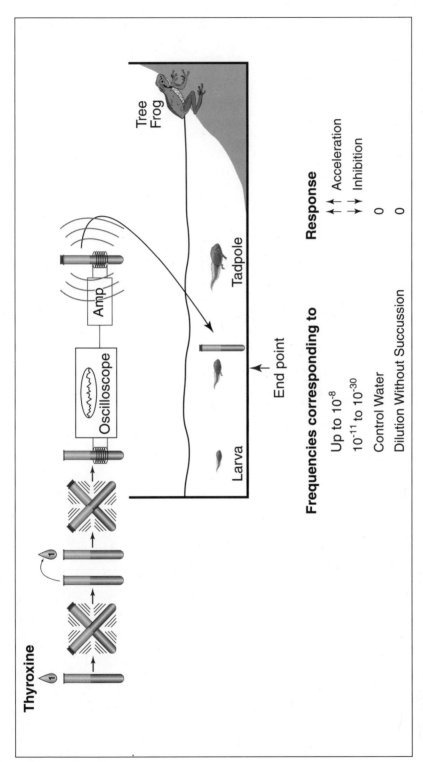

FIGURE 29 Digitized frequencies corresponding to potencies activities water in sealed glass vial which in turn modulates metamorphosis of tadpoles.

without thyroxine, and thyroxin dilutions without shaking had no effect.

In the next step, homeopathically prepared thyroxin dilutions were placed in a glass vial, which was in turn placed in the culture water. **The metamorphosis was inhibited without direct contact!** Clearly, some information was being transferred through the glass!

In the next step, electrical frequencies were acquired from a vial of potentized water surrounded by an input coil and amplified. The frequencies ranged from 0.1 to 10 MHz. These signals were digitized and transmitted to pure water (without thyroxin). When placed in the culture water, the **metamorphosis was again inhibited** in comparison with controls. Thus, the information transmitted was electromagnetic in nature and transmitted by means of water!

In a final corollary, larvae which had been exposed to excitatory material doses of thyroxin were later exposed to a succussed 10^{-8} preparation, **which was able to inhibit the previous stimulatory effect.** Thus, the isopathic principle was confirmed.

The clarity and implications of these studies are astonishing, indeed. It is important to recall that the results were duplicated in eight other respected centers (though, it should also be noted, with occasional but notable exceptions, which raise questions for further investigation). Once again, it is notable that this is the type of research currently being funded by the European Parliament.

Summary

Extensive research has been done on living animals as to the effects of both isopathic and homeopathic preparations. Fundamentally, the studies prove that homeopathic dilutions do act, even beyond Avogadro's number. More importantly, the actions are specific according to the Similia Principle. As an example, Bismuth doesn't detoxify Arsenic poisoning and vice versa.

Several details of physiological mechanisms involving neural transmission, endocrine communication, and immune stimulation are demonstrated, but no one mechanism on a physiological level is shown—obviously. Living organisms are highly complex and their functions cannot be reduced to a common ground.

However, at the level of water and its interactions with enzymes, cells, and tissues, it can be seen that more than just a lock-and-key mechanism are at work. Electromagnetic field interactions are shown by Schulte and Endler in their experiments on tree frog tadpoles. Highly reproduced results prove that homeopathic potencies are not merely molecules in water, but electromagnetic field vehicles with specific frequency complexes as well, and that they are transmissible through glass and directly to developing organisms.

Such research points the way to a new frontier in biology more closely related to biophysics than to molecular biology.

6

Modern Homeopathic Practice

eturning to the inquiring skeptic, a question may persist: "OK. There is scientific evidence that potencies work, but what assurance is there that the suffering patient will get the desired response?" Indeed, so many varieties of homeopathy are available these days that there is a need to discriminate quality.

Simple information transfer does not guarantee depth, subtlety, and sophistication. The analogy of digital communications is apt. There is a lot of wasted fluff on the Internet commingled with worthwhile educational, artistic, and scientific material. Music is similar—some tasteless, some sublime.

Homeopathic self-care books are ubiquitous in bookstores these days. They describe 30 to 50 remedies used typically in acute situations of injury or illness. The remedy pictures describe peculiarities and keynotes that make for fascinating reading. Parents and patients derive hope that knowledge of these remedies give them a measure of control over their health. Besides, homeopathy can do no harm and just might prevent a doctor's visit. Why not?

In its place, self-care books are generally harmless and may help during an acute crisis. A problem arises when the situation really needs medical attention to diagnose, say, a concussion or meningitis. Nevertheless, for routine colds and flus and bruises, simple over-the-counter (OTC) use of remedies is appropriate and helpful.

Acute conditions by definition are self-limited. Even if an incorrect remedy is given, no harm is done and the illness subsides on its own, regardless. Meanwhile, a real benefit is derived from trusting the body's own healing forces without turning to suppressive solutions. And familiarization with some remedies helps the process of homeopathic self-observation, a skill which comes in handy when visiting a trained homeopath.

Good examples of this type of prescribing are scattered throughout the sidebars in this book. *Arnica* is a remedy that is safe in virtually every case. Even in someone undergoing chronic, constitutional treatment, it is extremely rare for *Arnica* to interfere.

There is good reason for this fact, even by the Similia Principle. *Arnica's* unique vibration has to do with bruise-type injuries and shock. It is a remedy originally found as an herb alongside hiking trails. Hahnemann did provings of it because of its indigenous use for injuries.

There is not a great deal of individuality involved in simple bruises. A bruise is a bruise is a bruise. *Arnica* fits that vibration and therefore heals in most individuals, even in very severe cases of shock, head injury, and heart attack.

A corollary to this is that whenever the reaction to an injury is peculiar, *Arnica* probably will not work. For example, if someone has an injury and becomes hysterically anxious or angry, chances are another remedy will be needed because *Arnica* is more characteristically stoic, denying any problem. Even after a moderate amount of reading, a layperson can discern this homeopathic principle in action. Self-care books may well provide alternative ideas.

We are currently witnessing an explosion in the marketplace of OTC remedies that can be purchased in health food stores and even in drug stores. By and large the preparation of these remedies meet homeopathic standards and are effective when properly prescribed. They are homeopathically prepared if the name of the remedy on the label contains a "c" or "x" to designate whether the dilution factor is 1:100 or 1:10. Single remedies are preferable, of course, because these are how provings are made. Besides, components of mixtures probably interfere with one another. Of course, some knowledge must be applied in selecting the correct single remedy.

Unfortunately, the growing popularity of homeopathy encourages the commercial production of combination remedies. Labeled by diagnosis, a mixture of remedies are thrown into a formula which may or not have any homeopathic logic. The hope is that by chance a correct remedy will be included.

Combination remedies may work on occasion, but more often than not they sell because the complaint is self-limited in the first place. Homeopathic understanding is that once remedies are mixed together, the resultant vibration is not identical to the sum of the separate parts. It becomes an entity of its own, which may or may not work in a given case. The analogy here is like trying to enhance a musical experience by mixing together all six of Bach's Brandenburg concertos all at the same time.

Commercialization helps spread name-recognition for homeopathy, I suppose, but a drawback of combination remedies is that the public misapprehends the principle. Instead of homeopathic individualization, they advocate allopathic diagnosis-based prescribing.

A further problem follows the use of combinations for chronic diagnoses. When labels suggest cures for "Hypertension," "Anxiety," "Allergies," "Asthma," "Arthritis," "PMS," or "Headaches," the patient can be led away from needed effective treatment. Chronic conditions may be momentarily suppressed at best, but the opportunity of permanent cure will be lost if combinations are used.

Moreover, chronic administration of remedies without proper supervision can lead to the very provings which are the basis of homeopathy. When healthy volunteers do a proving, the remedy is given daily until symptoms arise; then the remedy is stopped so as to avoid "engrafting" effects of the proving permanently. Taking combination remedies repeatedly over a long time may have no effect at all, of course, but if there is an effect, it may engraft symptoms if taken indiscriminately. Over time, the very symptom picture one is trying to cure may be exacerbated.

Recently, following on the popularity of the anti-impotence drug Viagra, radio commercials have been touting a remedy called "Vigorex." Part of the selling point is its meeting the "exacting standards of the Homeopathic Pharmacopoeia." This illustrates another misapprehension of homeopathy. Regardless of its mode of preparation, any remedy aimed at a particular diagnosis and given to an entire population without individualization is by definition not homeopathic prescribing. The odds of such a product being effective are low because of the variety and subtleties of possible types of impotence. For every 10 people suffering from impotence, 10 different remedies are likely to be needed.

Aside from OTC applications of homeopathy, there are a few variations on methods of professional prescribing as well.

Many untrained practitioners attend weekend seminars to learn principles and remedy pictures to apply as an adjunct to their practices. This can be useful when acute prescribing is kept separate from chronic. Most such practitioners can be trusted to make this distinction, and such prescribing is very appropriate.

Exceptions are also notable, of course, so the consumer must be attentive to the level of training of the practitioner administering remedies.

A few decades ago, a German physician developed a technique of measuring electrical conductivity through acupuncture meridians by attaching electrodes to the tips of fingers and thumbs. Called a Voll machine, the technique is to observe a needle on a dial move up and down and settle at various rates. After appropriate training, the practitioner is able to make quite sophisticated and subtle diagnoses of inner pathological processes and causations—often with an accuracy surpassing conventional diagnostic techniques.

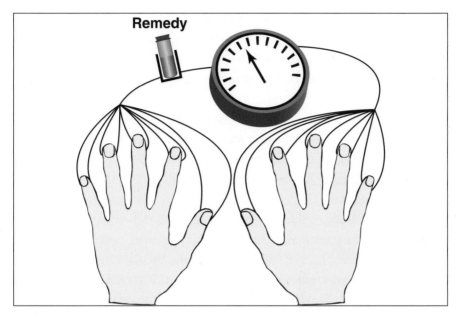

FIGURE 30   Diagram of the Voll machine measuring acupuncture meridians with a homeopathic remedy placed in the circuit ostensibly to balance the energy flow.

Used as a diagnostic tool, the Voll machine—and its more modern computerized counterparts—have a useful place in practice. A problem arises, however, when the same technique is used in treatment. Typically, substances, one by one, are placed in a well in the electric circuit to find one or more which will optimize the circuit. Most commonly, numerous single remedies are given to be taken on complex schedules over time. Frequent follow-up visits are scheduled to retest the circuits and change the formulations.

At a certain level, the Voll approach appears to duplicate the biophysical experiments described in Chapters 3, 4, and 5. Certainly some information is transmitted by this method, as it more closely approximates the Similia Principle than do OTC remedies. However, bandwidth issues remain, and dissonance rather than resonance are likely by relatively crude methods of frequency measurements.

Again, the analogy of music applies; viewing a symphony on an oscilloscope does not convey the same experience as listening to it. There is no obvious way to separate harmonic vs. dissonant vibrations. Merely playing a note of a certain frequency on a harmonica doesn't match the richness of that same note played on a cello or a French horn.

To fulfill the potential of homeopathy, extensive training is required—especially in treatment of chronic diseases. Not only is it necessary to master extreme subtleties of hundreds (even thousands) of remedy pictures, but the tremendous skill involved in case-taking is of paramount importance and requires years of practice and supervision. Even learning the complexities of modern homeopathic software demands considerable training and practice.

In my experience, training in classical homeopathy is far more demanding than medical school. The material itself is very extensive, but focussing on the whole person—mental, emotional, and physical—expands the character of the practitioner. The entire process must be free of bias while rigorously searching for truth. Extensive life-experience and personal growth are required to perceive correctly core issues and subtle distinctions that arise in nearly every interview.

Actually, the process of classical homeopathy is in many ways more demanding than other therapies of the patient as well. A great deal of unbiased self-observation is needed to get at the core issues with accuracy. A superficial "quick-fix" motive usually leads to a correspondingly superficial result. Patience is required as well, as it often takes several interviews before layers of compensation and rationalization and denial have been peeled away to reveal the central pathology.

Thus, the entire process is a quest for truth by both the practitioner and the patient.

When the process is successful, a picture emerges on all levels which is **coherent.** Homeopaths call it a symptom "totality." The remedy, which has been proven on volunteers and then macerated into solution and potentized, is administered on sugar granules. This

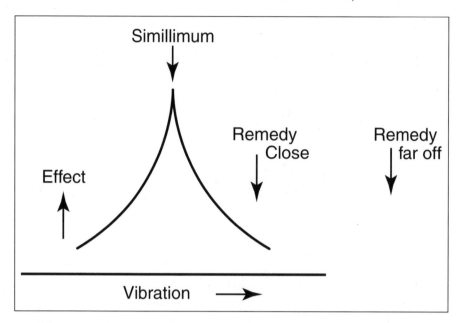

FIGURE 31   Resonance in regard to the effect of homeopathic remedies.

stimulates the healing forces of the patient through the principle of **resonance.** Over the ensuing weeks and months, the patient undergoes changes which follow known laws of cure.

Let us return to the principle of resonance again for a moment. An organism is made up of millions of individual frequencies—for each organic molecule, each enzyme, each subcellular organelle, each cell, each tissue, the muscles, the blood, the heart, the brain, each state of emotion, each thought, etc. The totality of frequencies combine into a coherent unity for the organism as whole. This then interacts with other organisms with greater or lesser intensity depending on resonance.

This can be depicted in a repeat of the resonance diagram, where the range of remedy frequencies is plotted against the energetic effect on the individual patient:

The aim is to find the substance in nature that most closely resembles the patient's totality.

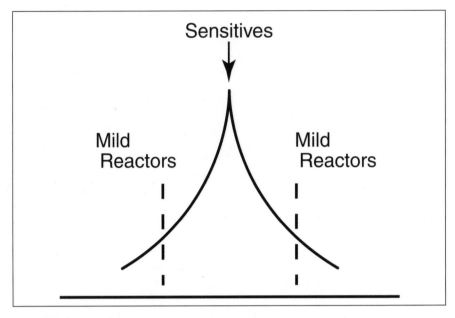

FIGURE 32   Resonance reactions in provers responding to a remedy being tested.

As described in Chapter 1, substances are tested on a population of volunteers. Some respond not at all. Many respond mildly, in vague ways. And a few are very sensitive to the substance, responding with striking, peculiar physical symptoms and elaborate, highly specific mental/emotional symptoms. The latter are most useful for matching to the patient. This may also be depicted by the same type of resonance diagram:

In this manner, provers are in a sense bio-meters for the remedy frequency.

Provers get homeopaths in the ballpark of remedy pictures. But their doses are stopped as soon as symptoms arise, so they cannot be pushed to the severity of symptomatology seen in patients with illness.

The next step in the evolution of a remedy picture is the collection of symptoms cured in cured cases.

Throughout history, some remedies came to be used more often than others—an inevitable consequence of the steep learning curve in homeopathy. Beginners know only a few remedies, so they tend to prescribe the same ones over and over. The knowledge base consequently tends to focus on a relatively small number of remedies.

The advent of computers is changing this tendency. After all, the virtual infinity of potential remedies in nature should all be useful. Computers enable us to search the massive database of known remedies and their symptoms in order to bring to the fore small remedies which might not be considered otherwise.

Recently, information about remedies has been gathered from metallurgical, botanical, and zoological sources. Just as plants and animals are categorizable into kingdoms and families, and minerals related via the Periodic Table of Elements, remedy pictures can be elaborated by similarities in their origins. Such analyses carry risk of unrealistic speculation which would only confuse or trivialize prescribing. On the other hand, they add rich dimensions to clinical or proving information.

The beauty of homeopathy is that it either works or it doesn't. The patient comes back better or the same. If the homeopath speculates about a remedy based on its botanical information, the hypothesis is confirmed in six weeks or so on follow-up. The feedback inherent in homeopathic practice makes clinical experience very valuable. It is well-grounded inquiry. . . . Perfect territory for a dedicated skeptic!

To illustrate just one level of subtlety that is common in practice: take the symptom "fear of cancer." This symptom is commonplace, especially in our culture. At first blush, it seems natural. However, to a homeopath it needs to be sorted out in more depth.

> It could mean—underneath—a fear of death.
> It could bring up childhood traumas of abandonment, of being all alone in the big, bad Universe.
> It might be a fear of loss of control—as symbolized by overgrowth of cells.
> It could represent a fear of being dependent or a burden on others—which in turn could point toward a pathological degree of independence.

129

Or perhaps it means a fear of being revealed as a coward in the eyes of others in the face of stress.

For some, it might signify their just due for past sins of diet, lifestyle, sex, or whatever.

For others, this symptom might be an obsessive-compulsive dwelling on a theme—which might be not only cancer, but money, family, work, etc.

For still another, it might simply be a sign of suggestibility—the idea may not have occurred except for a TV show depicting someone with cancer.

Each of the above interpretations represent different remedy possibilities. During the case-taking process, **every single symptom** is investigated in similar depth for subtlety. Eventually, a pattern emerges which lead to the **essence** of a case. Essence plus the coherent totality of the rest of the case—particularly considering the most peculiar aspects—make up the principal elements in remedy selection.

Finding a classical homeopath capable of carrying out such a process is not difficult. Usually, the label "Classical Homeopath" implies enough training to make the distinction. Having an MD degree is not necessary at all, although it sometimes helps in dealing with the medical system. There are a number of schools who train classical homeopaths, and they all entail three to four years of intensive work. The classroom portion may only be monthly, but the typical study load is about 30 hours/week! Not for dabblers!

Classical homeopaths schedule one hour or more for the initial interview, and usually a half hour or more for follow-ups. Generally, the interview entails a majority of attention focussed on the mental/emotional plane.

Finally, a single remedy is prescribed and six weeks to a few months will be taken for evaluating the average case. Of course, there are always exceptions to these general guidelines.

Follow-up itself is a whole other matter. Great skill and experience is involved in judging the action of a remedy. Some cases progress quickly to annihilation of the disease, and everyone agrees.

More often, however, a process is set in motion analogous to turning an ocean liner with a tug boat. Gradual changes occur in specific sequence, often cycling over weeks and months through various symptoms from the past. These usually are not intense in themselves, but patients often react to them with fear or despair. They can be seen as a regression. A little education suffices, and eventually a confidence grows that the body really is healing in an orderly fashion.

In retrospect, after months have passed, it is clear that a miracle has occurred. But in the midst of daily ups and downs that are normal, it can be hard to appreciate.

Practicing homeopathy is both a science and an art. There are sound, verifiable principles to follow. And there are also subtleties that flow without clear form—yet are real nevertheless.

Sometimes listening to a patient can be like I imagine painting a picture to be. I hear one thing and think I understand, but later information creates a paradox that needs to be resolved. If I can, I pursue that paradox until it clarifies itself. If I were a painter, I can imagine doing the nose over and over again until it is right. Settling for partial or imprecise understanding doesn't work. The subtlety of remedy vibrations requires precision to be truly effective.

Another analogy might clarify the concepts of coherent water and Information Theory:

One could take a case and hear B Flat in the patient's statement, "I am depressed." A generic remedy could be given for "depression," but the effect would be analogous to someone hearing a tone in the key B flat. It might resonate a little, but it is unlikely to produce a lasting response.

A more careful practitioner might inquire further and discover some of the circumstances of the depression—whether financial, romantic, or due to poor nutrition or lack of exercise. This might be analogous to finding a certain popular song, or some Muzac in B Flat. Again, only fleeting in effect.

A more experienced practitioner might find out about the personality of the patient—what is unique about his sensitivity to the circumstances that led to depression. This could be like deciding whether to offer the person a CD of something in B Flat by The Who or something from classical music.

Finally, a very insightful practitioner might touch on a core delusion, or a central meaning, that has driven the patient's entire perception of life. Here the distinction might be made between a Tchaikovsky Symphony in B Flat, a Beethoven in B Flat, or a Bach Contata. When the correct one is found, the inspiration is beyond the individual. The impact is deep and powerful—and lasting.

Summary

Research has certainly progressed to the point of rendering the mechanism of action of remedies rational and comprehensible. Once we have remedies, however, the task is to prescribe with quality. Homeopathy, when done correctly, is more than administration of a combination over-the-counter. It is more than connecting to acupuncture points and measuring superficial (though seductive) changes. It is a complex art that demands the full humanity of both the practitioner and the patient. They are partners in a quest for truth. Inherent in the process is a feedback that provides rapid reward when done accurately, and no result when applied imprecisely. As such, homeopathy is a rapidly evolving science and art that holds great promise in an era seeking powerful, nontoxic, and relatively inexpensive therapies for chronic disease.

Remedy Archetypes

Descriptions of remedies so far in this book have been very simplistic. The range and subtlety of remedy pictures in actual practice are profound—and always evolving as the profession grows.

For the beginning homeopath, the sheer volume of remedy pictures (2500 or so) is overwhelming. It is tempting to resort to memorization of "keynotes" and mnemonic trickery to hold seemingly disparate pieces of information together. Indeed, a certain amount of rote learning is necessary in the beginning to provide a foundation upon which to build.

As a homeopath gains clinical experience, patterns of personality types emerge for each remedy as patients come back cured. Of course, this can be a lengthy and painstaking process of observation.

Once a practitioner is well grounded in observing human beings and respectful of their variety and profundity—the master teachers in the world become a valuable resource. In my own development, I have been blessed by exposure to some of the great thinkers of the modern era—most especially my mentor and friend George

Vithoulkas—but also other influences, including Lou Klein, Rajan Sankaran, Massimo Mangialavori, Jan Scholten, Alize Timmerman.

This is just my limited list. There are many other master teachers in the world with vast experience. They each have their unique lens on human nature and of individual remedy pictures. The range is astounding, but the value of such teachings is that they powerfully inform individual practice. Time and again, when seated in front of a patient, he or she says something which rings a bell from something I have heard or read. That sparks a line of inquiry which very often leads to the remedy.

Ultimately, a homeopath must be steeped not only in books, but also in people. An inner reflection is developed into what really makes a given patient tick. The same process applies to learning remedies. It has been said that to truly know a remedy, one must live it for awhile—almost like an actor taking on a character.

If a homeopath has lived a remedy, the gait, manners of speech, choice of words, even the look in the eye become familiar. As this recognition dawns during the consultation, a symptom picture falls into place which matches a remedy picture known to the homeopath. He or she then asks questions about concrete confirmatory symptoms to ground the prescription and to guard against mere speculation.

The following brief descriptions of some remedy archetypes and some samples of corresponding cured cases from my practice hopefully provide a glimpse of the depth and humanness of homeopathy.

Nux vomica

Nux vomica, commonly known as "poison nut," is a member if the Loganiaceae family and has been known as a drug since 1540 A.D. The fruit of the tree is about the size of an orange and contains a bitter, gelatinous pulp. This pulp, it is said, is eaten by some of the birds of India, although it is well known to contain the poison Strychnine. The *Nux* itself is the seed deprived of the pulp and shell.

A wide variety of symptoms emerge from the provings, including muscle spasms, intestinal and uterine cramping, intense nausea and vomiting, headaches, chills, and insomnia. The full description would be too voluminous to include here.

The essence of the *Nux vomica* archetype is of an intense, hard-driving, **COMPETITIVE** personality characterized by anger and even rage. Especially male *Nux vomica* types live from one obstacle to another, relishing the challenge. They are often said to be driven to win at all costs, somewhat like Billy Martin (the Yankees manager). But I have found them to be mostly self-challenged, always setting the bar a little higher.

Nux vomica tends to be focussed on **EFFICIENCY.** They excel in professions like computers, sales, the military. They tend to be punctual and orderly in function, and concise and direct in speech. They like things to run smoothly. It is when things don't go well that they may blow up, often getting full of rage—swearing, yelling, slamming doors, punching walls, and sometimes fighting. Characteristically these outbursts of temper blow over quickly without resentment or grudges

They expect as much of others as they do of themselves, which leaves little room for imperfection. They operate well in corporate hierarchies, striving for the top more out of challenge than a true desire to win. *Nux* types may be harsh managers but often work well with people because getting along is more effective.

Nux vomica is frequently workaholic. They work long hours, then need instant relaxation. So they may drink heavily, smoke to excess, and utilize drugs to the extent of outright addiction. Their minds are so full of details and project challenges that sleep comes slowly and fitfully. Unfortunately, they are also very sensitive to noises, making sleep more difficult.

Generally the *Nux* body type is either thin and wiry, once again like Billy Martin, or stocky and square—like Pete Rose. Mentally they tend to be direct, frank, practical, and fact-oriented. Some might say they are very left-brained. The task is to "get the job done."

135

Interestingly, it is hard for *Nux vomica* to relax fully unless they are away on vacation with nothing else to do.

When under stress, *Nux* suffers stomach pains and even ulcers. A peculiarity is that muscle contractions work against themselves. Instead of vomiting freely, they go into spasm with "waterbrash" and nausea, or gas pains that are difficult to bring up. If constipated they have strong ineffectual urging. Even skeletal muscles tend to be "muscle bound" yet tight rather than flexible.

If sensitive to temperature *Nux* tends to be chilly rather than warm. They often dislike drafts or open air. Sun causes headaches and eyes are very sensitive to glare. For women, menstrual cramps are common and very intense.

Food cravings tend to be for coffee, alcohol, cigarettes, spices, and fatty meats. But they are often aggravated by these. It is frequently used as a routine antidote to drug toxicity and hangovers.

In later stages, as illness progresses they may collapse from exhaustion. Obsession with obstacles to challenge may eventually result in paranoid delusions—the idea that people are out to get them. In very extreme cases the tendency to rage can lead to homicidal impulses.

A nux vomica case

In 1992, I saw a patient I'll call Paul, a 30 year-old computer engineer with a wife and son. One year previously, while practicing "high falls" in Aikido, he developed pain in the right shoulder; initially this was thought to be tendinitis. Soon numbness developed on the inside of the right elbow. X-rays and MRI were inconclusive. The pain increased and spread to a disabling degree. Gradually he developed paralysis of his forearm, deltoid muscles, and even "winging" of the right scapula from atrophy. On examination, he showed severe atrophy of the entire right upper extremity. Of course, this severely impaired his job functioning.

The eventual neurological diagnosis was "Parsonage-Turner syndrome"—an acute brachial neuritis of unknown cause, although viral or immunologic inflammation was suspected.

The homeopathic interview revealed that the pain was originally "burning, stinging." He needed medication for severe spasticity of the right shoulder and arm. He got bronchitis easily with every cold. He was sensitive to cold in general.

At age 15–16, Paul had encephalitis but refused to tell anyone because he was intent on completing his school work. He got bored quickly if not working. He prided himself in being goal-oriented and rational, in doing his job very systematically. Thus he ended up having too many projects going at once.

Paul enjoyed Aikido because of the harmony he found competing with friends at his same level. He was sick with a virus yet continued training too hard because of being close to getting his brown belt. This injury is what led to the Parsonage-Turner.

Paul also had allergies. He desired spicy food strongly, and Coca-Cola moderately. He slept all right, though he highly valued his sleep. He usually slept with five blankets. He was very aggravated by cold drafts.

He enjoyed Aikido, but disliked swimming and running because they involved ending up back at the starting point.

Nux vomica 200, was given in one dose in Feb. 1992. All symptoms disappeared within a few weeks, and he regained full use of his arm.

Argentum nitricum

Argentum nitricum is silver nitrate, the same chemical salt used in infant's eyes at birth and to cauterize canker sores in the mouth. It has a very interesting place in homeopathic archetypes.

The essence of *Argentum nitricum* is a peculiar combination of **IMPULSIVITY** and **OBSESSION.** *Argentum nitricum* people are very passionate, animated, and excitable. They are performers by instinct, from a very early age. They feel things strongly, and they love to connect with people. It is not so much that they are show-offs, like *Lycopodium,* or covering an inner insecurity. They truly love to touch people emotionally, to share their innate excitability.

I used to teach this remedy by asking people to tune into a particular weatherman on TV. His quickness of mind and enthusiasm epitomized *Argentum nitricum.* Ironically, my hunch was later born out during a late-night TV interview in which he was the spokesman for a national phobia organization. He revealed that he had severe performance anxiety, a phobia of airplanes, and a peculiar fear of bridges over running water. These happen to be exact phobias belonging to *Argentum nitricum*. An additional phobia is of high places because of an uncontrollable impulse to jump.

This latter is a good example of the *Argentum nitricum* essence. When on a high ledge, they look over the side, and the impulse comes to jump. But in *Argentum nitricum* the impulse turns into an obsessive thought. They feel as if they are on the verge of being pulled over the edge. Suddenly, they **SNAP** to their senses, realizing they were momentarily insane, and in danger!

The peculiar quality in *Argentum nitricum* is the suddenness of the impulse and the catching of it later. One instance was of a man watching his son crossing the street to go to school. He suddenly had an image that a car would come around the corner and hit his son. Lost in this thought, he ran down the stairs and almost into the street before realizing how crazy this was!

It seems that these reflexive responses have to do with an excitability of the emotions and of the nervous system. They have anticipatory anxieties just looking forward to an event. This excitability may be so strong as to impact the nervous system. *Argentum nitricum* has a myriad of nervous system disorders—from multiple sclerosis to diabetic polyneuropathy, including various spasticities.

A common target organ for *Argentum nitricum* is the gastrointestinal tract. Canker sores (stomatitis), stomach ulcers, severe distension and flatulence, Crohn's disease, and ulcerative colitis respond to *Argentum nitricum*.

They tend to be very warmblooded and crave both sweets and salt equally. They startle easily and are sensitive to noise, light, odors, and intense emotional atmospheres.

An *Argentum Nitricum* Case of HIV
Carl is a 30 year-old gay man with a positive test for HIV, weakness, a weakened immune system, and a strong history of many griefs. Several courses of standard HIV therapy failed

because of side-effects, so he sought homeopathic care.

He tended to both excitability and depression. On the one hand, he was the life of the party, even publishing a newsletter of wild stories that entertained his neighborhood. On the other, he was easily embarrassed by small slips of the tongue at work, over which he obsessed for days and weeks into an isolated depression.

I treated him for about six months with an incorrect remedy and no response. Then he told me a story: he was cleaning snails out of his garden, heedlessly throwing them over his shoulder. It was during an era of racial rioting. A large black man was walking down the street. Just as my patient was tossing a snail over his shoulder, he realized someone was there but was too late to stop. He hit the black man right in the chest. He profusely, even obsequiously, apologized, but the man became irate nevertheless. Nothing happened in the end, but my patient obsessed over this for weeks. This story reminded me of *Argentum nitricum.*

He was given *Argentum nitricum* 1M, one dose, in Oct. 1992. His recovery was rapid and complete, to the point that even his friends have come for homeopathic treatment, commenting on their observation of his progress. (For the curious, his symptoms disappeared but he was not retested for HIV; because the antibody is an attempt on the part of the body to eliminate the virus, it would not be expected to turn negative in response to treatment).

Sulphur

The remedy *Sulphur* is made according to Hahnemann: from "Flowers of sulphur, Flores sulphuris, sublimed in fine acicular form into the receiver of a retort, washed by being shaken up with alcohol, in order to remove any acid that may be adhering to them." Hahnemann also explained in his Materia Medica: "Though sulphur has been employed for many centuries, by medical and non-medical persons, in the itch of workers in wool, yet none of them ever observed that the beneficial effects they saw from its use in the eruption of itch was effected by sulphur by similarity of action and homeopathy."

139

In homeopathy *Sulphur* is probably the most widely known of all remedies. It is used by many as a virtual specific for itchy skin eruptions, but in truth it needs to be individualized to the patient. Two basic archetypes are described: the classic "philosopher" type and what I like to call the "mechanic" *Sulphur* type.

The classic philosopher is typified as an absent-minded professor who is stoop-shouldered, shuffling around in open sandals, rather unkempt in appearance and disorderly in his environment. He is enamored of his own ideas, constantly theorizing about abstract concepts in a wide variety of conceptual realms. The classic image is of an inventor trying to create the first perpetual motion machine which requires no energy. He has disdain for mundane issues such as hygiene, chores, finances, even relationships. His skin is dirty-looking, often smelly, and itchy.

The "mechanic" *Sulphur* is not so commonly described in books but is seen often in practice. This person, whether male or female, is robust, plethoric, very frank and practical-minded. Men are often immersed in inventive mechanical projects, whereas female *Sulphurs* are very involved in raising children in creative ways. These people are highly opinionated, full of life, and often alcoholic.

These images are classic and often helpful, but in practice we see a wide variety of types—from computer engineers to waitresses, from businessmen to yoga instructors. Often the remedy is found purely on physical symptomatology, which might include itchy skin aggravated at night and in the heat of bed, general aggravation and perspiration in heat, catnap sleep while sticking feet out from under the covers, smelly foot sweat, and craving for sweets and the fat on meat while disliking eggs. Body type varies from lean and stooped to obese and plethoric. They tend to be sloppy (although sometimes extremely neat), and frequently have a fear of heights.

The inner essence is very distinct in *Sulphur* but somewhat difficult to describe. They do tend to **THEORIZE** a lot and typically are very confident in their opinions. A unique quality is the ability to see things from many perspectives at once. They can argue any side of an issue, even though they have their own strong opinion. A *Sulphur* person is able have an opinion and simultaneously see his own prejudices, so despite having an unshakable faith in his own perspectives on things there is also a kind of humility. *Sulphur* is thus very complex but usually quite intellectual.

One characteristic that is consistent in *Sulphur* is **EGOTISM.** Though they can see their own hangups clearly, they nevertheless rarely lack self-confidence. The egotism is so inherent that even when wrong, the point is that it is *their* perspective. Nobody else can quite understand.

Therefore the vulnerability in *Sulphur* patients is when they are **UNAPPRECIATED.** For *Sulphur,* relationships are mutual self-appreciation contracts. It is true that some *Sulphur* patients do not need to be appreciated in the moment, but they know that they will be someday—perhaps even after death. So, many are artists or composers, inwardly focussed on creativity, but nevertheless holding onto the idea that they will one day be "discovered."

A *Sulphur* Eczema/Leprosy Case

In 1993, I saw Jayesh, a 30 year-old computer engineer born originally in India. He suffered from eczema for 18 months and had tried steroids without success. He scratched to the point of bleeding, mostly in the evening and after showering. At the age of 12–13 he had leprosy, which was treated with antibiotics.

Very hardworking, Jayesh typically did the work of two employees in his highly competitive computer company, trying hard to earn money to support a house and his family. He always tried to be the best at whatever he did; it was a matter of pride for him. It was hard for him to relax, as he always worried about the future, which he considered an unknown that was difficult to control. Even watching sporting events caused him anxiety because he tried so hard to anticipate the outcome mentally. His mind is always trying to solve puzzles—three solutions to a software problem may come to him in his sleep.

Jayesh craved sweets and ice cream strongly, as well as spicy and sour foods. Basically he was vegetarian by cultural background, though he never really craved meat. He had an aversion to eggs. His itching was worse from the heat of bed, so he put his leg out of the covers even though his extremities tended to be cold. He was always very sloppy, hated bathing. He perspired on the soles of his feet especially at night. He also had dandruff, which itched considerably.

He had a severe head injury at age 11, then became very solitary because of the injury and the leprosy, which affected the scalp.

In February 1993, Jayesh was given *Sulphur* 1M, one dose. What ensued was fairly typical for skin eruptions in deep cases. His eczema spread over his arms and legs and exuded a yellow discharge which lasted for several months. He was determined to get well without steroids, which were clearly suppressive and not curative, so he waited even in spite of entreaties from family and co-workers.

Finally, the eczema subsided to a spot on the scalp where he used to have the leprosy. This eventually developed a horny growth which was very noticeable at exactly the location of the leprosy on his scalp! In addition, the nerves in his arm which were damaged by the leprosy came to life again, causing choreic movements reminiscent of when he had antibiotic treatment. This all disappeared over a span of months.

One year after the remedy, he was completely cured except for a small patch of eczema on his leg which arose under the stress of his father's death. There has been no recurrence since.

Thuja occidentalis

Thuja is the Arbor Vitae conifer, a tincture made from fresh green twigs prior to potentization.

The core essence of *Thuja* is a very common story in society, but hard to elicit in the interview. Their story begins in childhood with neglect, or sometimes outright abuse. Often there is alcoholism or mental illness which occupies the focus of attention, a constant crisis mode which does not allow children to be free and emotional. They are required to be seen, not heard. For survival it becomes important to learn to **FIT IN**, to not stand out or attract attention.

Boys learn to be proper and obedient. Girls learn to be pretty and charming. Conformity is the goal of life.

As teenagers they make a detailed, systematic study of how to behave. They observe the walk, the gestures, the speech, the make-up that work for other people. They become geniuses at mimicking others. As adults they can be the best salesperson, spouse, parent, church-goer—fitting in perfectly everywhere. They are so skilled that they become chameleons socially. They can fit in in a wide variety of circumstances. I have seen *Thuja* act curatively in actors, motor-cycle gang members, even people with purple hair, but the common denominator is the desire to fit in with whatever crowd they belong to.

DECEIT is a common theme for *Thuja*, not merely in the sense of outright lying but more in being selective while sharing information. *Thuja* people tend to tell only what is minimally necessary in the moment. Their lives become compartmentalized; one set of friends know certain things while others know entirely different aspects. To *Thuja*, this is the way life is for everyone—so they may not describe it as pathology in the interview.

A lifetime of living in the *Thuja* manner results in a person who has no real sense of identity inside. They may be able to say the right thing for the right moment, but it is hard for them to know what they really think and feel as individuals. As a consequence, *Thuja* people have an inner sense of being **UNLOVABLE.** They suspect that any-one who would know them for real would not love them, or find them attractive. I recall one person from Hollywood, a stunningly beautiful woman, who admitted she had always felt unattractive inside.

This state is not exactly one of "low self-esteem" as it is neu-tral. *Thuja* has so little self-sense that they don't actively put them-selves down. Instead, their self-sense is one of invisibility. They act a part but don't feel present.

On the physical plane, *Thuja* patients tend to be bothered most by cold damp weather. They frequently manifest tumors, growths,

143

and particularly warts. Chronic sinus drainage or vaginal discharge are common. Stomach troubles, intestinal cramps, ovarian pains, left-sided headaches, arthritis of all types are presenting reasons for coming to a homeopath. Peculiarly, they are often intolerant to onions and garlic. Also, offensive foot sweat may occur.

Case of Self-destructive Depression

Jasmine, a 40 year-old single woman had been in psychotherapy for 12 years for depressions; at her worst, she carved her forearms with self-hating words. From childhood she was brought up to take blame for anything bad that happened; for example, if a dog dies she believes it is because of the dog food she made for it. Even success was viewed as a jinx that will lead to disaster.

As a child she was very shy, had no friends. Her parents did not want children but had three. Her mother hated her laugh and warned her against having any fun. As a teenager she was incredibly naive about sex and found boys who tried to rape her. Eventually she felt dogs were her best friends, perhaps even her only friends. She describes herself as always making herself into what others want her to be.

Physically she suffered chronically from stomach aches and bladder pains whenever she was upset. She was chilly, chronically constipated, and intolerant to raw onions.

Initially I gave *Aethusa* and considered *Staphisagria*, but she did not improve until *Thuja* 1M in 1988, after admitting she felt "unlovable" since being sent away by her parents at age 3. She underwent considerable improvement month by month, then had a setback when her sister died of a brain tumor. Homeopathic *Ignatia* 1M helped her through this crisis. Years later, she did very well with *Silica* 1M and 10M as a next layer.

Carcinosin

Most homeopathic remedies are made from plants or minerals, but occasionally they are made from human disease tissue. *Carcinosin* is prepared from human cancer tissue, neutralized of course, and then shaken and diluted beyond Avogadro's number. It is unique among remedies in that it was used at first in a cancer clinic without formal provings. Its image has to this day been derived primarily from clinical experience.

Carcinosin is another remedy arising from childhood neglect and/or abuse. Originally found in families of cancer patients in which crisis was normal, it is nowadays found in families with alcoholism, drug addiction, mental illness, and violence. The idea is similar to *Thuja's* invisibility, but the *Carcinosin* story is more of learning to take care of everyone. From a young age they try to maintain peace and order, taking care of details others miss in the midst of crisis. Rather than having a playful childhood, *Carcinosin* patients develop an adult-level sense of responsibility. If anything at all goes wrong, they take it personally.

Throughout life *Carcinosin* becomes a classic "**CO-DEPENDENT**." They place the needs of others over their own, to an extreme degree. Frequently the homeopathic interview is taken up primarily by the problems of family members or friends than by the patient's concerns. It can be difficult to elicit the patient's own story.

Control is a common story in *Carcinosin*. They tend to be fastidious, often punctual, and have hawk-like eyes over tiny details that could potentially spiral out of control. Like spouses of alcoholics, they make great efforts to present a positive picture to the outside world, even though inner life is chaotic.

Carcinosin can be very busy and hurried, and they tend to be compulsive about vigorous exercise. As children, they love to dance. This persists into adulthood, along with hiking. Many modern authors emphasize *Carcinosin's* love of nature and animals.

Carcinosin people tend to be warmblooded if anything, though not strikingly so. Usually they may be markedly better by the seashore, although sometimes worse. Typically there is a strong desire for chocolate, often fruit, sometimes salty foods or meat.

The Case of a Harassed Caretaker

Alice is a 70 year-old pleasant and vital lady in a difficult situation. After a long and satisfying marriage producing children, now grown and quite successful in their own ways, she finds herself in a situation from which she cannot extract herself. Her husband fell on ill health, suffering from several severe health conditions. Once very active, he became very limited in activities, gradually housebound, and finally confined to bed. Alice took on the tasks of caring for him, fighting with Medicare, arranging nursing, etc.

At first, out of love and caring, she took the burdens on willingly. But her husband's decline was long and lengthy. She found herself with no life of her own. From her first waking thought to her last before falling to sleep, her focus of attention was on her husband's needs. Much of this was of necessity, but during homeopathic consultation she had to admit that she had really lived this way all her life.

I had treated Alice for many years with various remedies, as had other homeopaths before me. Finally, it dawned that this was a case of classic Codependency. It became clear that the anxiety and stress symptoms she exhibited—palpitations, fatigue, insomnia, and even food allergies and sinusitis—derived from this inner pathology. She did not have a life of her own because she could not.

Carcinosin 200 brought about a gradual but definite improvement in her outlook, energy, and symptomatology. Over ensuing years, her husband's health declined, and he finally died. She maintained her improved outlook, found new friends and activities, and regained her strength in spite of the inevitable stress.

After his death, Alice did well for awhile, but gradually fell back into old patterns of depression, self-pity, fear of the future, etc. Another dose of *Carcinosin* 1M pulled her out of that state. At last notice, she had a circle of friends, new interests, and is an avid golfer.

Calcarea carbonica

Calcarea carbonica is "calcium carbonate" but is derived from an inside scraping of an oyster shell grown in a pollution free environment.

Calcarea, along with *Sulphur*, is one of the most common remedies in the entire materia medica of 2500 remedies. In early stages of relative health, the *Calcarea* person is highly responsible, worka-holic, very practical, and reliable. From childhood they pride them-selves in being **FUNCTIONAL** and capable. They also tend to be systematic in their approach to learning or in tackling problems. Unlike *Nux vomica*, *Calcarea* people tend to work too hard not out of a sense of challenge but out of responsibility. They are the "salt of the earth" people to whom others turn for reliable outcomes. They find it hard to say "no" when a task is important.

Over time *Calcarea* types take on too much and become **OVER-WHELMED.** They generally have strong constitutions and can han-dle a lot, but there is a limit. Then they become fatigued, anxious in the midst of their overwhelm, averse to any work at all, and very fear-ful about the future. They cancel their schedules and just hibernate until they can recuperate.

Because they are fundamentally strong in constitution, *Calcarea* tends to be a common remedy at the extremes of age—in children because they are still strong, and in the elderly who have self-selected themselves by surviving so long without developing other layers of pathology.

There are two basic body types: lean and wiry, and "fair, fat, and flabby." In either case they are innately hardworking type peo-ple. Typically they are full of anxieties, mostly about functioning. Hence, they worry about the future, about poverty, about crippling illness, about losing their mental functioning, about being a burden on others. They are not particularly fastidious but rather systematic and plodding.

Physically, *Calcarea* tends to be chilly, especially in cold damp weather. They perspire easily, most often on the scalp, back of the neck, and feet, as well as the face and upper lip with minimal exer-tion. In bed at night, they tend to sleep on the left side; they go to bed with socks on, but have to take them off later because their feet become too hot. Food cravings are typically for sweets, often eggs (especially soft-boiled or poached), and sometimes salty food or meat. They have vertigo from high places, and often fear spiders and mice.

Disease categories for which *Calcarea* cures range from hypo-
or hyperthyroidism, fibromyalgia, arthritis, hypoglycemia, chronic
fatigue syndrome, constipation, colitis, hypertension, heart failure,
headache, vasculitides, and many others.

A Case of Grave's Disease

Laila was a 44 year-old accountant, originally from India. She
was very healthy until 1989, when she found her mother after
she had had a stroke, she had lost her job after having overworked
10 hours/day 7 days/week, and lived in fear of a neighbor bran-
dishing a gun. She began losing weight rapidly despite a large
appetite. Despite fear and fatigue, she persisted in working too
hard. Finally she developed tremors, lost hair, and developed
heart palpitations. A physician diagnosed hyperthyroidism
(Grave's Disease) with a radioiodine uptake of 64% (normal
25–35%), T4 of 7.0 (normal 0.7–1.9), and TSH < 0.03 (normal
0.5–4.5).

She craved sweets strongly. Used to gain weight easily, and was
chilly, until developing hyperthyroidism. She always felt highly
responsible for others. Her characteristic nature was to control
her emotions so as to be able to function. She was always very
independent and self-sufficient. She had a fear of poverty and
homelessness.

She was given *Calcarea carbonica* 200, one dose, in June of
1991. Within 6 weeks, she regained energy and weight, her pulse
had reduced to normal, and she was much less anxious. By April
1991 her TSH was 0.9 (normal 0.5–4.5). In Aug. 1992, the TSH
was still 2.4. The last follow-up was Summer of 1997, and she
continued to do well.

Sepia

Sepia is made from the brownish-black ink of the cuttlefish, which
is used to evade predators. The fable is that Hahnemann first proved
this remedy after noticing the poisoning effects of painters licking
their brushes.

The homeopathic uses of *Sepia* are myriad. It is classically used
in females, particularly in relation to hormonal changes such as

menarche, menopause, PMS, in nausea of pregnancy, postpartum depression, and after abortion. However, it is frequently useful in men as well.

The inner essence of *Sepia* has to do with **APATHY**—an inner stagnation of nervous and endocrine systems leading to an emotional state of indifference. When we are healthy, the neuroendocrine systems are actually in a state of imbalance which defines our gender and attraction between sexes. In hormonal states, the imbalance becomes nullified, creating a state which is unnatural and stagnant. This can become a state of *Sepia* pathology.

In *Sepia* the core apathy can be so great that it manifests as clinical depression. There may be a lack of affection, even a revulsion to sex. A classic situation is being pregnant and looking forward to having children, only to feel resentment and hatred for the husband and child after delivery. The woman feels as if the spiritual realm of love has forsaken her, and that there can be no cure for her lack of feeling. Also, a keynote is "weeping without cause" which is probably really a reflection of a despair that they can be helped at all.

Only a few things stimulate her out of her apathy—anger, exercise, and stimulants. It seems that conflict leading to anger will activate feelings; then she is able to feel love and even sexuality. Exercise has the same effect if it is vigorous. *Sepia* also craves stimulants such as coffee, cigarettes, and pungent spicy, sour foods, and chocolate to help stimulate feelings.

At the peak of pathology, *Sepia* patients can be very bitchy—shrieking, screaming, even violent. At the same time, the emotional apathy lends itself to frankness and penetrating intelligence. This can become sarcastic, but it can also be insightful in situations of business, marketing, or politics.

Generally *Sepia* patients are chilly, especially in the extremities. Their symptomatology tends to be left-sided and worse from 3 to 5 PM. They tend to be nauseated (especially in hormonal circumstances) and have constipation which manifests as a lack of urge for days on end.

A Depression Case

Rachel, a 36 year-old physical therapist, came for treatment in 1992. She suffered from left-sided migraines, homesickness for her home country of Argentina, severe insomnia, and fatigue. All this began soon after her daughter was born three years previously.

Her husband was hospitalized with endocarditis, but she felt little about that. She dwelled on uncontrollable thoughts of suicide. She was indifferent to patients, didn't wish to keep her house clean, and didn't care whether the children took their baths. She worked out regularly at a fitness center, but awoke nightly at 3 a.m. trying to decide whether to divorce her husband and go back to Argentina. She described herself as being very changeable, weeping for no reason, and yelling constantly especially at her kids.

She had irregular periods, left-sided sciatica before menses, and was very chilly in general. She craved sweets, chocolate, and coffee. She had a persistent fear that something bad would happen to her kids.

She was given *Sepia* 1M, one dose, in April 1992. Another dose was given a year later, but she continued to do extremely well until November 1997, at which time she needed one more dose.

Veratrum album

Veratrum album is the white-flowered Hellebore. N.O. Melanthacae (of the Liliaceae), made as a tincture of the root-stocks collected (in the Alps and Pyrenees) early in June before flowering.

As a remedy it has both acute and chronic uses. As an acute remedy it is often given in cholera with severe explosive diarrhea, chills, and profuse perspiration with extreme thirst for cold drinks, lemons, and a tendency to chew on ice.

Constitutionally *Veratrum* applies in hyperactive, wound-up individuals who are always busy, but aimlessly so. They do repetitive activities, but accomplish nothing, and are often loquacious. It can be a major remedy in ADHD; it is as if the neurons in the brain are disconnected, resulting in scattered dyslexic thinking.

One of the major themes psychologically is an intense struggle for self-esteem, but peculiarly focussed on a feeling of inferiority/superiority in social hierarchies. They either in actuality have been born into the upper crust of society, or they imagine they have. As life goes on, there is constant class comparisons, even to the point of racism or chauvinism. Often, however, they find themselves in relatively menial occupations, always dreaming with envy of what they think they should have attained.

Anger is very prominent in *Veratrum,* to the point of rage. They can be violent, or at least threatening, but not as destructive as a number of other remedies. In *Veratrum* this arises from a true nervous system state, a kind of neurotransmitter imbalance, rather than because of a psychodynamic process.

Veratrum people often are chilly, but may ignore the cold. They tend to be quick, scattered, and intense. Food cravings tend to be be for lemons, salt, and cold drinks, even to the point of loving to chew ice.

In the same way, *Veratrum* can be easily frightened. Ailments from fright, affecting the nervous system, are common. Common diseases are neurological conditions, colitis, and urological problems.

In late stages, *Veratrum* can become virtually psychotic. A graphic picture is of a rambling preacher on a cold streetcorner beseeching everyone to repent. Fright, rage, and arrogance are characteristic in this stage.

A Case of Autism

In April 1995, a 4 year-old child was brought to me with a diagnosis of autism made at UCLA from the age of 20 months. In the office, she was obsessed by the fan, the heater grate, and barely looked at me. She had had tantrums from birth. She had severe insomnia, waking frequently to drink water and from night terrors. Her breath smelled like sweet beer.

Her speech stalled at age 2. From 11 months of age she constantly flipped through the pages of books for 5 hours a day. At 2½ months of age, she was frightened whenever people laughed in her presence. She let out piercing screams upon visiting people's houses. Peculiarly, she masturbated at just a few years of age.

She was always very thirsty, ate dirt and bugs, chewed on ice, and loved lemons. She ground her teeth.

Veratrum album 200 was given. Within 2 days she was potty trained, which had been a chronic problem. Within 2 months UCLA confirmed considerable improvement. She was less obsessive in all ways. She no longer ate ice, dirt, or bugs.

Within 7 months she had made such gigantic strides in mental development that she was entered in kindergarten. She was shy but independent. She had no fears or tantrums. She was soon discharged as well by UCLA.

Summary

As in previous discussions about resonance and the complexity of remedies, the pictures themselves are fascinating and multi-faceted. The task of a homeopath is both an art and a science, necessitating sound knowledge of memorized "keynotes" but also the breadth and subtlety of each individual human picture. To get results, the individual patient and the unique remedy must be known deeply. Approximations fail. Nevertheless, the very human nature of the process is enlivening in itself.

Implications and Challenge for the Future

As in physics, the focus of research in biology is gradually changing from the purely structural and chemical focus to an emphasis on quantum electrodynamics as the basis for biophysical phenomena. This shift has profound implications for homeopathy, because the Principle of Similia and the method of potentization can now be understood and validated.

Researching the role of electrodynamic interactions will undoubtedly become a primary activity for not only homeopathy—but for allopathic drug companies as well. Many allopathic drugs may have subtler actions than mere chemical effects. The uniqueness of individual reactions to medicines is becoming accessible to research. Not only might such reactions become more predictable, but the sensitivity of individuals might even be exploited for benefit.

Avogadro's number—once a stumbling block to imagining a mechanism—can now be seen clearly as irrelevant. Clustered, coherent water is stable, replicates itself, and is a very capable transmitter of complex and subtle information.

At last, homeopathy as a method can stand secure on understanding of mechanisms. Standardizing of remedies will be an immediate outcome. Cataloguing the natural resonant frequencies of substances in nature will provide a foundation for research with powerful implications for the future.

Perhaps the creation of such foundations will encourage funding for more research, as is already happening in the National Center for Complementary and Alternative Medicine of the NIH, and the European Committee for Homeopathy of the European Union.

Clarifying the mechanisms involved in Similia and Potentization hopefully will improve accuracy and effectiveness of homeopathic prescriptions. Methods of delivering kinetic energy to water may be developed which will enhance the power of potencies.

An immediate practical advantage of accurately detecting and measuring remedies is that they can be standardized. Potencies from different pharmacies may be compared. Effects of exposure to sunlight, heat, and aromatic odors, not to mention electromagnetic fields themselves, can be tested. Pharmacies may be able to more accurately test for impurities. Even the place for combination remedies conceivably could be clarified.

Furthermore, electrodynamic studies of people before and after taking remedies might add to our understanding of the details of mechanisms of action. It is known that coffee, camphor, mothballs, tea tree oil, electric blankets, and dental drilling can antidote remedies, at least temporarily. How these occur is completely unknown. Perhaps now it is amenable to investigation.

As techniques for measuring electrodynamic fields of patients and remedies improve, the slowness of empiricism may give way to greater and swifter precision.

The discovery that information can be transmitted by electromagnetic frequencies is intriguing, to say the least. The concept that remedy vibrations can be digitized and transported by CD or the Internet is mind-boggling. Even so, it is my opinion that this will ultimately have little impact on the conduct of practice. In order to maintain their full richness, digitized remedies will always need to be prepared at their origin by high quality pharmacies, even if those pharmacies shift over time to transmitting their remedies digitally. Practitioners will require the same degree of training and skill to prescribe with precision.

Information theory itself is still in its infancy, and this book does not do it justice. Concepts of holographic transmission, fractal phenomena, and chaos theory are emerging as analogies at the least, and perhaps deeper mathematical truths in reality. In this context, Hahnemann's precise development of the Principle of Similars may be truly prescient. The Similia principle could well represent a more general principle of resonance in nature.

For homeopathy, great strides are being made in the conduct of provings. The methods utilize the objectivity of placebo-controls. Dreams are being regarded as fruitful sources of information. Most especially, the most sensitive people are being selected in advance as provers so that the full remedy picture can be elucidated in more detail. Finally, provings are beginning to be videotaped, so that subtle expressions of provers can be observed by homeopaths, which adds immensely to the ability to perceive it in patients.

Public Policy Implications

A potentially important benefit of increased funding by government agencies may be the generation of cost-benefit studies. Preliminary impressions are that considerable money could be saved by utilizing homeopathy, especially in the treatment of chronic conditions. Not only is treatment relatively inexpensive, but its duration is shortened by the curative outcome.

If this turns out to be true when rigorous cost-benefit analyses are done, insurance companies and managed care systems might benefit greatly. The consequence of this might alter the relationships between homeopaths and allopaths. Already the *New England Journal of Medicine* article seems to have softened opinions toward

155

homeopathy, [Eisenberg DM, *et al,* 1993] so greater cooperation can be anticipated.

How might this look in practice?

To put the situation in context, costs of the medical/pharmaceutical industry have been rising at an alarming rate—to the point that governmental officials, politicians, and major industrial leaders are aggressively attempting to control costs. Debates over managed care and insurance coverage caps rage continually.

One way of viewing the managed care crisis is to look carefully at underlying assumptions. The definition of health used in homeopathy—viewing the person holistically rather than as a system of specialized parts—is a legitimate, common-sense yardstick for measuring outcome. If our medical system were operated based upon this holistic principle, the overall health of the population would be improved optimally, and very likely at considerably less cost.

A natural outcome of cost-benefit analyses and public policy adjustments would be to recognize homeopathy as a legitimate specialty within the medical system, as has been done very successfully in many countries. In part this is already happening.

Homeopathy is specifically licensed in four states as of this writing—Connecticut, New York, Arizona, and Nevada. It is recognized as a legitimate subspecialty of Naturopathy in 12 states. Having been written into the Food and Drug Act of 1937, it is accepted in every state as a legitimate practice by otherwise licensed practitioners.

There are also changes in attitudes within the medical profession itself. When I first began practice in the early seventies, there was frank derision toward homeopathy. In recent years I have seen open interest expressed in medical meetings and respectful comments made to patients.

Cooperative professional interaction does not require full belief in homeopathy—merely respect for it as a profession in its own right. After all, psychiatrists and surgeons coexist despite wide differences in worldview.

What role might homeopathy play in the medical system of the future? A homeopath is an appropriate specialist to see for preventive medicine and many aspects of family practice. He or she might be the first to see people with chronic disease, trying a nontoxic approach first before resorting to treatments requiring benefit/risk judgment calls.

Even in allopathic terms the homeopathic point of view could be a useful balancing perspective. Dr. Garcia-Swain's research on alcoholics/addicts in recovery is an excellent model for this blending of systems.

Homeopathy would be an especially appropriate referral for patients in whom a diagnosis cannot be established. Homeopathy's advantage derives from its individualizing the remedy to the uniqueness of the patient's symptoms, bypassing the need for diagnosis altogether.

A particular value in accepting homeopathy as a specialty could be collaboration in research. Research listed herein demonstrates the practicality of such collaboration. There are challenging paradoxes yet to be investigated. However, the tools are improving dramatically as of just the last few years.

Perhaps the most important challenge is in the realm of education. Children could be taught from a young age to understand the meaning of symptoms as signs of the body trying to heal and to have faith in the body's ability to heal. Naturally, respect for serious signs must be taught as well, but the overall focus of health education should shift from fear-based to health-enhancing preventive orientations.

Moreover, medical education itself might benefit from a homeopathic perspective. Basic medical sciences and diagnostic techniques need not change much, but a holistic perspective would help de-fragment the specialties. In a sense, this is already occurring in modern medical schools which are using modular approaches— patient-based learning to integrate all the specialties at once. Homeopathy and its individualized focus fit nicely into this milieu.

The bottom line needs to be a clear conception of what constitutes a whole person in true health. This vision is held firmly as a standard for every homeopath during every interview with every patient. It is inherent in the very mind-set. The promise for patients as individuals—and society as a whole—is freedom from chronic disease evolving from a nontoxic, powerful, and natural method of healing.

Glossary

Allopathy: A term for orthodox or standard medicine. Based on the roots *allo-* meaning *other,* and *pathos* meaning *suffering.* Refers to counteracting symptoms as being a problem needing suppression.

Avogadro's Law: equal volumes of all gases and vapors at the same temperature and pressure contain the same number of molecules. A way of comparing dissimilar molecules by creating a standard. A "Gram Molecular Weight" of one substance contains the same number of molecules as a "Gram Molecular Weight" of another substance, the weight of which is characteristic for each substance.

Avogadro's Number: 6.0220943×10^{23}. molecules in a Gram Molecular Weight. A dilution beyond 10^{-24} represents the point in serial dilution beyond which there is no molecule of the original substance left. This dilution would look like this if done in one action: 1/ 1,000,000,000,000,000,000,000,000

Chaos: Seemingly disorderly patterns in the Universe which on investigation have properties definable mathematically.

Classical Homeopathy: the homeopathic method using a single substance to treat the whole person (mental, emotional, and physical) and then allowing time to allow the healing.

Clathrates: expanded clusters of water enclosing smaller clusters inside of which are replications of the original structure which duplicate its specific shape.

Clusters in water: specific alignments of water molecules under the influence of electromagnetic fields possessing stability and ability to replicate themselves in random water.

Coherence: molecules moving in a coordinated fashion within electromagnetic waves with well-defined relative phases compared to random water. Also applies to tissues and crystals with molecules aligned in similar coordinated fashion in relation to an electromagnetic field.

Engrafting: the ability of homeopathic remedies on sugar granules to transmit their potency to unmedicated granules.

Fractal: a characteristic produced mathematically and found in nature in which the same patterns are found in microscopic subsets of macroscopic patterns. In this way information signals are carried in small structures as well as in large structures.

Gram Molecular Weight: The weight of a standard number of molecules (Avogadro's Number) of any given substance.

Homeopathy: A 200 year-old system of therapy based on stimulating the body to heal itself by stimulating it by the Similia Principle. From the roots *homoio-* meaning *similar,* and *pathos* meaning *suffering.*

I_E Water: clustered water as developed by Dr. Shui-Yin Lo.

Isopathy: a principle of therapy using the identical substance which causes symptoms. From the roots *iso-* meaning *identical,* and *pathos* meaning *suffering.*

Mole: One Gram Molecular Weight.

Plussing: the ability of potentized water to transmit its potency to unmedicated water.

Potentization: a process of serial dilution and succussion of a solution, thereby increasing its effectiveness as a homeopathic remedy when prescribed according to the Similia Principle.

Proving: the systematic process of administering a homeopathic remedy to a group of volunteers and carefully recording symptoms so as to discover the curative properties of that substance.

Quantum Electrodynamics: mathematical perspectives applying to submolecular and atomic interactions based on Einsteinian relativistic concepts as opposed to chemical principles of interaction.

Resonance: Transference of energy between two substances vibrating with identical frequencies. The closer the vibrations, the more energy is transferred. Close frequencies transfer less energy. Frequencies far apart from one another transfer undetectable energies.

Resonant frequency: The optimal frequency of vibration of a particular substance, tissue, organ, or organism.

Similia Principle: The homeopathic Law of Similars. *A substance which produces a spectrum of symptoms in a healthy will cure that spectrum of symptoms in a sick person.* Based on the concept of resonance.

Succussion: shaking of a solution in the process of potentization.

Vital force: the principle defined by Samuel Hahnemann as underlying the activities of all living organisms, possessing innate intelligence for maintaining homeostasis.

References

Adey WR (1988) Physiological signalling across cell membranes and cooperative influences of extremely low frequency electromagnetic fields. In: *Biological Coherence and Response to External Stimuli*. Frohlich H (ed) Springer-Verlag. Berlin. p. 148.

Aissa J, Litime MH, Attias E, Allal A, Benveniste J (1993) Transfer of molecular signals via electronic circuitry. *FASEB J*. 7: A602 (3489).

Albertini H, Goldberg W (1986) Evaluation d'un traitement homéopathique de le néuralgie dentaire. Bilan de 60 observations dentaires in recherches en homéopathie. *Fondat. Franc. Rech. Homéopath*. Lyon p. 75.

Alberts B, Bray D, Lewis J, Raff M, Roberts K, Watson JD (1989) *Molecular Biology of the Cell. 2nd Edition*. Garland Publ. New York.

Albrecht-Buehler G (1991) Surface extension of 3T3 cells towards distant infrared light sources. *J. Cell. Biol*. **114**: 493.

Amodeo C, Dorfman P, Ricciotti F, Tétau M, Veroux PF (1988) Evaluation de l'activité d'Arnica 5CH sur les troubles veineux après perfusion prolongée. *Cah. Biother*. **98**: 77. Quoted in Bellavite and Signorini (1995).

Anagnostatos GS (1994) Small Water Clusters (Clathrates) in the Homeopathic preparation Process in Endler and Schulte, 1994.

Arani R, Bono I, Del Giudice E, Preparata G (1995) *Int. J. Mod. Phys*. **B9**: 1813.

Aubin M (1984) Elements de pharmacologie homéopathique. *Homéopathie Française* 72: 231. In: Bellavite P and Signorini A (1998) *Fundamental Research in Ultra High Dilution and Homeopathy.* Kluwer Academic Publishers, Dordrecht. p. 65.

Bastide M, Aubin B, Baronnet S (1975) Etude pharmacologique d'une preparation d'Apis mel. (7CH) vis-à-vis de l'erytheme aux rayons U.V. chez le cobayes albinos. *Ann. Hom. Fr.* 17 (3): 289. Reported in: Bellavite P and Signorini A (1995) *Homeopathy: A Frontier in Medical Science.* North Atlantic Books, Berkeley. p. 58.

Bastide M, Doucet-Jaboeuf M, Daurat V (1985) Activity and chronopharmacology of very low doses of physiological immune inducers. *Immunol. Today* 6: 234–235.

Bastide M, Daurat V, Doucet-Jaboeuf M, Pelegrin A, Dorfman p. (1987) Immunomodulatory activity of very low doses of thymulin in mice. *Int. J. Immunotherapy* 3: 191–200.

Bastide M (1994) Immunological examples on ultra high dilution research. In: Endler PC and Schulte J (eds) *Ultra High Dilution.* Kluwer Acad. Publ. Dordrecht. p. 27.

Bastide M, Boudard F. (1995) A novel concept of immunomodulation, Guenounou M (Ed) *Forum sur l'Immunomodulation,* John Libbey Publishers, Paris. pp. 303–316.

Baumans V, Bol CJ, Oude Luttikhuis WMT, Beynen AC (1987) Does Chelidonium 3x lower serum cholesterol? *Brit. Hom. J.* 76: 14–15.

Beauvais F, Bidet B, Descours B, Hieblot C, Burtin C, Benveniste J (1991) Regulation of human basophil activation. I. Dissociation of cationic dye binding from histamine release in activated human basophils. *J. Allergy Clin. Immunol.* 87: 1020.

Bellavite P, Chirumbolo S, Signorini A, Bianchi I (1991b) Effects of various homeopathic drugs on superoxide production and adhesion of human neutrophils. *5th GIRI Meeting.* Paris, Abs. 1

Bellavite P and Signorini A (1995) *Homeopathy: A Frontier in Medical Science.* North Atlantic Books, Berkeley.

Bellavite P and Signorini A (1998) *Fundamental Research in Ultra High Dilution and Homeopathy.* Kluwer Academic Publishers, Dordrecht. p. 105.

Bellavite P and Signorini A (1998) Biological effects of electromagnetic fields. In: Schulte J and Endler PC (Eds.) (1998) *Fundamental Research in Ultra High Dilution and Homoeopathy.* The Netherlands: Kluwer Academic Publishers. p. 127.

Benveniste J, Arnoux B, Hadji L (1992) Highly dilute antigen increases coronary flow of isolated heart from immunized guinea pigs. *FASEB J.* 6: A1610.

Benveniste J, Aissa J, Litime MH, Tsangaris GTh, Thomas Y (1994b) Transfer of the molecular signal by electronic amplification. *FASEEB J.* 8 (4): Abs. 2304.

Bildet J, Guyot M, Bonini F, Grignon MC, Poitevin B, Quilichini R (1990) Demonstrating the effects of Apis mellifica and Apium virus dilutions on erythema induced by U.V. radiation on guinea pigs. *Berlin J. Res. Homoeopathy* 1: 28.

Bildet J, Dupont H, Aubin M, Baronnet S, Berjon JJ, Gomez H, Manlhiot JS (1981) Action in vitro de dilutions infinitésimales de Phytolacca Americana sur la transformation lymphoblastique à la phytohemagglutinine. *Ann. Hom. Fr.* 23 (3): 102. In: Bellavite P and Signorini A (1995) *Homeopathy: A Frontier in Medical Science.* North Atlantic Books, Berkeley.

Boiron J, Cier A (1962a) Elimination provoquée et specifité d'action des dilutions infinitésimales d'élements toxiques. *Ann. Hom. Franc.* 4: 789–795. Reported in: Schulte J and Endler PC (Eds.) (1998) *Fundamental Research in Ultra High Dilution and Homoeopathy.* The Netherlands: Kluwer Academic Publishers. p. 196.

Boiron J, Cier A (1962b) Recherches expérimentales d'une activité isopathique. *Ann. Hom. Franc.* 10: 796–800. Reported in: Schulte J and Endler PC (Eds.) (1998) *Fundamental Research in Ultra High Dilution and Homoeopathy.* The Netherlands: Kluwer Academic Publishers. p. 196.

Boiron J, Marin J (1967) Action de dilutions homéopathiques d'une substance sur la cinétique d'élimination de cette même substance au copurs de la culture de grains prálablement intoxiqués. *Ann. Hom. Fr.* **9:** 121–130. Reported in: Schulte J and Endler PC (Eds.) (1998) *Fundamental Research in Ultra High Dilution and Homoeopathy.* The Netherlands: Kluwer Academic Publishers. p. 197.

Boiron J, Cier A, Vingert C (1968) Effects de quelques facteurs physiques sur l'activité pharmacologique de dilutions infinitésimales. *Ann. Hom. Franc.* **10:** 187–196. Reported in: Schulte J and Endler PC (Eds.) (1998) *Fundamental Research in Ultra High Dilution and Homoeopathy.* The Netherlands: Kluwer Academic Publishers. p. 196.

Boiron J, Abecassis J, Belon P, Cazin JC, Gaborit J (1978) The effects of Arsenicum album 7CH upon rats poisoned with arsenic-quantitative study and statistical value of the results. *Proc. 35th Hom. Congress.* pp. 1–18.

Bonavida B (1992) TNF and TNF Receptors: Structure, mechanism of action and role in disease and therapy. *Drugs of Today,* Vol. **28.**

Bonavida B, Safrit Jt, Miorimoto H (1993) Reversal of drug resistance: Synergistic Anti-Tumor Cytotoxic Activity by combination treatment with drug and TNF or toxins. *Cancer Therapy,* 75:169–176.

Bonavida B, Gan XH (1998) Induction and Regulation of Human Peripheral Blood TH1-TH2 Derived Cytokines by I_E Water Preparations and Synergy with Mitogens. In: Lo SY, Bonavida B (eds) *Proceedings of the First International Symposium on Physical, Chemical and Biological Properties of Stable Water [I_E™] Clusters.* World Scientific, Singapore.

Bordas J, Diakun GP, Diaz FG, Harris JE, lewis RA, Lowy J, Mant GR, Martin-Hernandez ML, Towns-Andrews E ((1993) Two-dimensional time-resolved X-ray diffraction studies of live isometrically contracting frog sartorius muscle. *J. Musc. Res. Cell. Mot.* **14**: 311–324.

Both G (1987) Zur prophylaxe und therapie des metritis-mastitis-agalactie (MMA)—komplexes des schweines mit biologischen arzneimitteln. *Biologische Tiermedizin* **4**: 39. Reported in: Bellavite P and Signorini A (1995) *Homeopathy: A Frontier in Medical Science.* North Atlantic Books, Berkeley. p. 58.

Boyd WE (1954) Biochemical and Biological Evidence of the Activity of High Potencies. *Brit. Hom. J.* **44**: 7–44.

Brigo B (1987) Le traitment homéopatique de la migraine: une étude de 60 cas, controlée en double aveugle. *Journal of Liga Med. Hom. Int.* **1**: 18.

Brigo B, Serpelloni G (1991) Homeopathic treatment of migraines: A randomized doubleblind controlled study of sixty cases. *Berlin J. Res. Homeopathy* **1** (2): 98.

Bullock TH (1997) Electromagnetic sensing in fish. *Neurosci. Res. Program. Bull.* **15**: 17.

Cal JC, Larue F, Guillemain J, Cambar J. (1986) Chronological approach of protective effect of *Mercurius Corrosivus* against mercury induced nephrotoxicity. *Ann. Rev. Chronopharmacol.* **3**: 99–103.

Cal JC, Catroux P, Dorfman P, Cambar J. (1988a) Variations saisonnières de l'action du mercure et du platine en homéopathie expérimentale. *GIRI* **27**: (Abs.). Reported in: Schulte J and Endler PC (Eds.) (1998) *Fundamental Research in Ultra High Dilution and Homoeopathy.* The Netherlands: Kluwer Academic Publishers. p. 197.

Cal JC, Larue F, Dorian C, Guillemain J, Dorfman P, Cambar J. (1988b) Chronobiological approach of mercury-induced toxicity and of the protective effect of high dilutions of mercury against mercury-induced nephrotoxicity. *Liver Cells and Drugs.* **164**: 481–485.

Callens E, Debiane H, Santais MC, Ruff F (1993) Effects of highly dilute beta2-adrenergic agonists on isolated guinea pig trachea. *Brit. Hom. J.* 82: 123.

Cambar J, Desmouliere A, Cal JC, Guillemain J. (1983a) Mise en évidence de l'effet protecteur de dilutions homéopathiques de mercurius corrosivus vis-à-vis de la mortalité au chlourure mercurique chez la souris. *Ann. Hom. Fra.* 5: 6–12. Reported in: Schulte J and Endler PC (Eds.) (1998) *Fundamental Research in Ultra High Dilution and Homoeopathy.* The Netherlands: Kluwer Academic Publishers.. p. 197.

Cambar J, Desmouliere A, Cal JC, Guillemain J. (1983b) Influence de l'administration de dilutions infinitésimales de mercurius corrosivus sur la mortalité induite par le chlorure mercurique chez la souris. *Bull. Soc. Pharmacol. Bordeaux* 122: 30–38. Reported in: Schulte J and Endler PC (Eds.) (1998) *Fundamental Research in Ultra High Dilution and Homoeopathy.* The Netherlands: Kluwer Academic Publishers. p. 197.

Cazin JC. (1986) Etude pharmacologique de dilutions hahnemanniennes sur la rétention et la mobilisation de l'arsénic chez le rat. In: Boiron J, Belon P, Hariveau E: Recherche en Homéopathie. Fondation Francaise pour la Recherche en Homéopathie. pp. 19–39. Reported in English: Schulte J and Endler PC (Eds.) (1998) *Fundamental Research in Ultra High Dilution and Homoeopathy.* The Netherlands: Kluwer Academic Publishers. p. 196.

Cazin JC, Casin M, Gaborit JL, Chaoui A, Boiron J, Belon P, Cherruault Y, Papapanayoutou C (1987) A study of the effect of decimal and centesimal dilutions of arsenic on the retention and mobilization of arsenic in the rat. *Human Toxicol.* 6: 315–320.

Cazin JC, Cazin M, Chaoul A, Belon P (1991) Influence of several physical factors on the activity of ultra low doses. In: Doutremepuich C (ed) *Ultra Low Doses.* Taylor and Francis, London. p. 69.

Chan KYG, Inal F, Senkan S. (1998) Suppression of Coke Formation in the Steam Cracking of Akanes: Ethane and Propane. *Proceedings of the First International Symposium on Physical,*

Chemical and Biological Properties of Stable Water [I$_E$] Clusters. Singapore: World Scientific Publishing, p. 105.

Chaoul A (1988) Influence de certains facteurs physiques et chimiques sur l'activité de dilutions infinitésimales d'arsénic. Thesis. Univ. Lille Fac de Pharm.

Chez AR, Jonas WB (1997) The challenge of complementary and alternative medicine. *Amer. J. Obstetrics & Gynecology* **177**: 1156–1161.

Chirila M, Hristescu S, Manda G, Neagu M, Olinescu A (1990a) The action of succussed substance on the proliferative response of human lymphocytes in vitro stimulated with phyto-haemaglutinin. In: *Proc. 4th GIRI Meeting,* Paris, Abs. 11

Chirila M, Hristescu S, Manda G, Neagu M, Olinescu A (1990b) The action of succussed substance on the proliferative response of human lymphocytes in vitro stimulated with phyto-haemaglutinin. In: *Proc. II Congr. Int. OMHI,* Ediciones Tecnico Cientificas, Mexico, p. 23.

Chirumbolo S, Signorini A, Bianchi I, Lippi G, Bellavite P (1993) Effects of homeopathic preparations of organic acids and of minerals on the oxidative metabolism of human neutrophils. *Brit. Hom. J.* **82**: 237.

Cier A, Boiron J, Vingert C, Braise J (1966) Sur le traitement du diabéte expérimental par des dilutions infinitésimales d'alloxane. *Ann. Hom. Fr.* **8**: 137. Reported in: Bellavite P and Signorini A (1995) *Homeopathy: A Frontier in Medical Science.* North Atlantic Books, Berkeley. p. 58.

Colas H, Aubin M, Picard P, Lebecq JC (1975) Inhibition du test de transformation lymphoblastique (TTL) à la phytohemag-glutinine (PHA) par phytolacca americana en dilution homéopathiques. *Ann. Hom. Fr.* 17 **17** (6): 629. In: Bellavite P and Signorini A (1995) *Homeopathy: A Frontier in Medical Science.* North Atlantic Books, Berkeley. p. 72.

Conforti A, Signorini A, Bellavite P (19933) Effects of high dilutions of histamin and other natural compounds on acute inflammation in rats. In: Bornoroni C (ed) *Omeomed 92* Editrice Compositori, Bologna, p. 163.

Coulter H (1982).*Divided Legacy:Volume III. The Conflict Between Homoeopathy and the American Medical Association..* Second Edition. Berkeley: North Atlantic Books.

Daurat V, Dorfman P, Bastide M (1988) Immunomodulatory activity of low doses of interferon a, b in mice. *Biomed &Pharmacother.* **42:** 197.

Davenas E, Poitevin B, Benveniste J (1987) Effect on mouse peritoneal macrophages of orally administered very high dilutions of silica. *Eur. J. Pharmacol.* **135:** 313. Quoted in: Bellavite P and Signorini A (1998) *Fundamental Research in Ultra High Dilution and Homeopathy.* Kluwer Academic Publishers, Dordrecht. p. 67.

Davenas E, Beauvais F, Amara F, Robinson M, Miadonna A, Tedeschi A, Pomeranz B, Fortner P, Belon P, Sainte-Laudy J, Poitevin B, Benveniste J (1988) Human basophil degranulation triggered by very dilute antiserum against IgE. *Nature* **333:** 816.

Day C. (1986) Clinical Trials in Bovine Mastitis. *The British Homoeopathic Journal* 75: 11–14

De Caro G, Gentili L, Lucentini P (1990) Isoproterenol induced salivary gland enlargement is influenced in the rat by ultradiluted solutions of eldeisin. In: *Proc. 4th GIRI meeting.* Paris. Abs. 23.

De Gerlache J, Lans M (1991) Modulation of experimental rat liver carcinogenesis by ultra low doses of the carcinogens. In: Doutremepuich C (ed) *Ultra Low Doses.* Taylor and Francis, London. p. 17.

Delbancut A, Dorfman P, Cambar J (1993) Protective effect of very low concentrations of heavy metals (cadmium and cisplatin) against cytotoxic doses of these metals on renal tubular cell cultures. *Brit. Hom. J.* **82:** 123.

Del Giudice E, Preparata G, Vitiello G (1988) Water as a free electric dipole laser. *Phys. Rev. Lett.* **61:** 1085–1088.

Del Giudice E, Preparata G. (1998) Coherent Electrodynamics in

Water. *Fundamental Research in Ultra High Dilution and Homoeopathy* (Eds. Schulte J and Endler PC). The Netherlands: Kluwer Academic Publishers.

Dorfman P, Lasserre MN, Tétau M (1987) Préparation à l'accouchement par homéopathie. Expérimentation en double insu versus placebo. *Cah. Biother.* **94**: 77. Quoted in Bellavite and Signorini (1995), p. 47.

Doucet-Jaboeuf M, Guillemain J, Piechaczyk M, Karouby Y, Bastide M (1982) Evaluation de la dose limite d'activité du Facteur Thymique Sérique. *C.R. Acad. Sci.* **295**: III. In: Schulte J and Endler PC (Eds.) (1998) *Fundamental Research in Ultra High Dilution and Homoeopathy.* The Netherlands: Kluwer Academic Publishers. p. 230.

Doucet-Jaboeuf M, Pelegrin A, Cot MC, Guillemain J, Bastide M (1984) Seasonal variations in the humoral immune response in mice following administration of thymic hormones. In: Reinberg A, *et al*, (eds) *Ann Rev. Chronopharmacology* Vol.1. Pergamon Press, Oxford, p. 231.

Doucet-Jaboeuf M, Pelegrin A, Sizes M, Guillemain J, Bastide M (1985) Action of very low doses of biological immunomodulators on the humoral immune response in mice. *Int. J. Immunoparmacol.* **7**: 312.

Doutremepuich C, De Sèze O, Anne MC, hariveau E, Quilichcii R (1987) Platelet aggregation on the whole blood after administration of ultra low dosage Acetylsalicylic Acid in healthy volunteers. *Thrombosis Research,* **47**:373–377.

Doutremepuich C, De Sèze O, Le Roy D, Lalanne MC, Anne MC (1990) Aspirin at very low dosage in healthy volunteers: effects on bleeding time, platelet aggregation and coagulation. *Haemostasis.* **20**: 99–105.

Doutremepuich C, Aguejouf O, Pintigny D, Serillanges MN, de Sèze O (1994) Thrombogenic properties of ultra-low-dose of acetylsalicylic acid in a vessel model of maser-induced thrombus formation. *Thromb. Res.* **76**:225–229.

Eid P, Felisi E, Sideri M (1994) Super-placebo ou action pharmacologique? Une etude en double aveugle, randomisée avec un remède homéopathique (Caulophyllum Thalictroides) dans le travail de l'accouchement. *Proc.V Congr. O.M.H..I.,* Paris, 20–23. Quoted in Bellavite and Signorini (1995)

Eid P, Felisi E, Sideri M (1993) Applicability of homoeopathic Caulophyllum thalictroides during labour. *Brit. Hom. J.* 82: 245.

Eisenberg DM, Kessler RC, Foster C, Norlock FE, Calkins CR, Delbanco T. (1993) Unconventional medicine in the United States: prevalence, costs and patterns of use. *N Engl J Med.* 328: 246–252.

Elia V, Niccoli M (1999) Thermodynamics of extremely diluted aqueous solutions. *Annals NY Acad Sci* 879, 241–48.

Endler PC, Heckmann C, Lauppert E, Pongratz W, Alex J, Dieterle D, Lukitsch C, Vinattieri C, Smith CW, Senekowitsch F, Moeller H, Schulte J. The metamorphosis of amphibians and information of thyroxin storage via the bipolar fluid water and on a technical data carrier; transference via an electronic amplifier. *Fundamental Research in Ultra High Dilution and Homoeopathy.* The Netherlands: Kluwer Academic Publishers. 1998: p. 155.

Endler PC, Schulte J (1994) *Ultra High Dilution. Physics and Physiology.* Kluwer Academic Publishers, Dordrecht (The Netherlands).

Ferley JP, Zmirou D, D'Adhemar D, Balducci F (1989) A controlled evaluation of a homeopathic preparation in influenza-like syndromes. *Brit. J. Clin. Pharmac.* 27: 329.

Fisher p. (1998) The Information Medicine Hypothesis. *Fundamental Research in Ultra High Dilution and Homoeopathy* (Eds. Schulte J and Endler PC). The Netherlands: Kluwer Academic Publishers. p. xiii.

Fougeray S, Moubry K, Vallot N, Bastide M (1993) Effect of high dilutions of epidermal growth factor (EGF) on in vitro proliferation of keratinocyte and fibroblast cell lines. *Brit. Hom. J.* 82: 124.

Friese KH, Kruse S, Ludike R, and Moeller H. (1997) *Intl . J. of Clin. Pharm. Therapeutics.* 35

Friese, KHY, Kruse S, Moeller H. (1997) Acute otitis media in children: a comparison of conventional and homeopathic treatment. *Biomedical Therapy* 15: 113–122.

Frohlich H (ed) (1988) *Biological Coherence and Response to External Stimuli.* Springer-Verlag, Berlin.

Gaborit JL (1987) Etude pharmacologique de la rétention et de la mobilisation de l'arsénic sous l'effet de doses infinitésimales d'arsénic. DEA Pharmacochimie univ. Lille Ii Fac de Pharm.

Garcia-Swain S (1997). Thesis for Hahnemann College of Homeopathy. Soon to be published in two-volume textbook on addiction medicine.

Gibson RG.(1960) Homeopathic Therapy in Rheumatoid Arthritis: Evaluation by Double-Blind Clinical Therapeutic Trial. *British Journal of Clinical Pharmacology* **9**, 453–459.

Guillemain J, Cal JC, Desmoulières A, Tetau M, Cambar J (1984) Effet protecteur de dilutions homéopathiques de metaux néphrotoxiques vis-à-vis d'une intoxication mercurielle. *Cah. Biothérapie* 81 (suppl.): 27. In: Bellavite P and Signorini A (1998) *Fundamental Research in Ultra High Dilution and Homeopathy.* Kluwer Academic Publishers, Dordrecht. p. 75.

Guillemain J, Douylliez C, Bastide M, Cambar J, Narcisse G (1987) Pharmacologie de l'infinitésimal. Application aux dilutions homéopathiques. *Homéopathie* 4: 35. In: Bellavite P and Signorini A (1998) *Fundamental Research in Ultra High Dilution and Homeopathy.* Kluwer Academic Publishers, Dordrecht. p. 75.

Hahnemann S (Ed. Wenda Brewster O'Reilly) (1996). *Organon of the Medical Art.* 1842 . Redmond, WA: Birdcage Books.

Ho MW, Lawrence M (1993) Interference colour vital imaging—a novel noninvasive technique. *Microscopy and Analysis* 9: 26.

Ho MW (1995) *Neural Network World* 5: 733–750.

Ho MW (1998) Bioenergetics and the coherence of organisms. In: Schulte J and Endler PC (eds). *Fundamental Research in Ultra*

High Dilution and Homoeopathy. The Netherlands: Kluwer Academic Publishers. p. 69

Ho MW and Popp FA, Warnke U (1994) *Bioelectrodynamics and Biocommunication.* World Scientific, Singapore.

Hornung J (1991) An overview of formal methodology requirements for controlled clinical trials. *Berlin J. Res. Homeopathy* 1 (4/5): 288.

Jacobs J.(1994) Treatment of Acute Childhood Diarrhea With Homeopathic Medicine: A Randomized Clinical Trial in Nicaragua. *Pediatrics:* **93**: 719–725.

Jonas WB, Fortier AF, Heckendorn DK, Nacy CA (1991) Prophylaxis of tularemia infection in mice using agitated ultra-high dilutions of tularemia-infected tissue. In: *Proc. 5th GIRI Meeting,* Paris, Abs. 21.

Khuda-Bukhsh AR, Banik S (1991) Assessment of cytogenetic damage in X-irradiated mice and its alteration by oral administration of potentized homeopathic drug, Ginseng D200. *Berlin J. Res. Homeopathy* 1 (4/5): 254.

Kleijnen J, Knipschild P, Ter Riet G. (1991) Clinical trials of homoeopathy. *British Medical Journal.* **302**: 316–323.

Kolisko L (1926) Physiologischer und physikalischer Nachweis der Wirksamkeit kleinster Entitöten bei sieben Metallen. Goetheanum Vererlag, Dornach, Schweiz. In: Schulte J and Endler PC (Eds.) (1998) *Fundamental Research in Ultra High Dilution and Homoeopathy.* The Netherlands: Kluwer Academic Publishers.

Kremer F, Santo L, Poglitsch A, Koschnitzke C, Behrens H, Genzel L (1988) Coherence of low-intensity millimeter waves on biological systems. In: *Biological Coherence and Response to External Stimuli.* Frohlich H (ed). Springer Verlag, Berlin. p. 233

Lapp C, Wurmser L, Ney J (1955) Mobilization de l'arsenic fixé chez le cobaye sous l'influence des doses infinitésimales d'arseniate. *Therapie.* **10**: 625. Reported in: Bellavite P and Signorini A (1995) *Homeopathy: A Frontier in Medical Science.* North Atlantic Books, Berkeley. p. 58.

LaRue F, Cal JC (1985) Mise on évidence de l'effet protecteur de différentes dilutions de mercurius corrosivus. *Cahiers de Biothérapie.* **88:** 71–78. Reported in Schulte J and Endler PC (Eds.) (1998) *Fundamental Research in Ultra High Dilution and Homoeopathy.* The Netherlands: Kluwer Academic Publishers. p. 197.

LaRue F, Cal JC, Guillemain J, Cambar J (1985) Influence du facteur dilution sur l'effet de mercurius corrosivus vis-à-vis de la toxicité induite par le chlorure mercurique chez la souris. *Hom. Fra.* **73:** 375–380. Reported in: Schulte J and Endler PC (Eds.) (1998) *Fundamental Research in Ultra High Dilution and Homoeopathy.* The Netherlands: Kluwer Academic Publishers. p. 197.

LaRue F, Cal JC, Guillemain J, Cambar J. (1986) Influence de la durée de prétraitement sur l'effet de mercurius corrosivus vis-à-vis de la toxicité induite par le chlorure mercurique chez la souris. *Hom. Fra.* **5:** 275–281. Reported in: Schulte J and Endler PC (Eds.) (1998) *Fundamental Research in Ultra High Dilution and Homoeopathy.* The Netherlands: Kluwer Academic Publishers. p.197.

Lauppert E (1995) Auswirkung von 'homöopathisch' zubereitetem Kupfersulfat auf das Wachstum von Weizenkeimlingen. Thesis, Graz. In: Schulte J and Endler PC (Eds.) (1998) *Fundamental Research in Ultra High Dilution and Homoeopathy.* The Netherlands: Kluwer Academic Publishers.

Linde K, Clausius N, Ramirez G, Melchart D, Eitel F, Hedges LV, and Jonas WB. (1997) Are the clinical effects of homoeopathy placebo effects? A meta-analysis of placebo-controlled trials. *The Lancet.* **350:** 834–843.

Litime MH, Aissa J, Benveniste J (1993) Antigen signaling at high dilution. *FASEB J.* **7:** A602 (3488).

Lo SY. (1996) Anomalous State of Ice. *Modern Physics Letters* **B10:** 909–919.

Lo SY, Lo A, Chong LW, Tianzhang L, Hua LH, Geng X. (1996) Physical Properties of Water with I_E Structures. *Modern Physics Letters* **B10:** 921–930.

Lo SY and Bonavida B. (1998) *Proceedings of the First International Symposium on Physical, Chemical and Biological Properties of Stable Water [I_E] Clusters* . Singapore: World Scientific Publishing.

Lo SY. Talk to National Center for Homeopathy, San Diego, CA. 1998.

Lo SY (1996) *Modern Physics Lett.* **B19:** 909–919.

Lo SY, Lo A, Chong LW, Tianshang L, Hua LH, Geng X (1996) *Modern Physics Lett.* **B19:** 921–930.

Monro J (1987) Electrical sensitivities in allergic patients. *Clin. Ecol.* **4:** 93.

Netien G, Graviou E, Marin M (1965) Action de doses infinitésimales de sulfate de cuivre sur des plantes préalablement intoxiquées par cette substance. *Ann. Hom. Franc.* **7:** 248–252. Reported in: Schulte J and Endler PC (Eds.) (1998) *Fundamental Research in Ultra High Dilution and Homoeopathy.* The Netherlands: Kluwer Academic Publishers. p. 197.

Noiret R, Glaude M. (1976) Etude enzymatique du grain de froment ontoxiqué par du sulfate de cuivre et traité par différentes dilutions hahnemanniennes de la même substance. *Rev. Belg. Hom.* **IX**(1): 461–495. Reported in: Schulte J and Endler PC (Eds.) (1998) *Fundamental Research in Ultra High Dilution and Homoeopathy.* The Netherlands: Kluwer Academic Publishers.p. 197.

Oberbaum M, Markovitz R, Weissman Z, Kalinkevits A, Bentwich Z (1992) Wound healing by homeopathic silica dilutions in mice. *Harefuah* **123:** 79–82.

Oberbaum M, Weisman Z, Markovitz R, Kalinkovich A, Bentwich Z (1991) Wound healing by homeopathic dilutions of silica in experimental animals. In : *Proc. 5th GIRI Meeting,* Paris, Abs. 23.

Oberbaum M, Markovitz R, Weisman Z, Kalinkevitz A, Bentwich Z (1992) Wound healing by homoeopathic Silicea dilutions in mice. *Harefuah (J. Israel Med. Ass.)* **123:** 78.

Palmerini CA, Codini M, Floridi A, Mattoli P, Buffetti S, Di Leginio

E (1993) The use of Phosphorus 30 CH in the experimental treatment of hepatic fibrosis in rats. In: Bornoroni C (ed) *Omeomed92.* Editrice Compositori, Bologna, p. 219.

Paterson, J (1944) Report on Mustard Gas Experiment. *J. Am. Inst. Homeopathy* 37: 47.

Pennec JP, Aubin M (1984) Effect of aconitum and veratrum on the isolated perfused heart of the common heel (Anguilla-anguilla) *Comp. Biochem. Physiol.* 776: 367.

Pennec JP, Aubin M, Manlhiot JL, Payreu B, Scaliger D (1984a) Action de differentes dilutions de veratrine sur le coeur isolé et perfusé d'anguille. *Homéopathie Française* 72: 245. In: Bellavite P and Signorini A (1998) *Fundamental Research in Ultra High Dilution and Homeopathy.* Kluwer Academic Publishers, Dordrecht. p. 65.

Pennec JP, Aubin M, Manlhiot JL, Payrau B, Scaliger D (1984b) Action de différentes dilutions de veratrine sur le coeur isolé perfusé de rat. *Homéopathie Française* 72: 251. In: Bellavite P and Signorini A (1998) *Fundamental Research in Ultra High Dilution and Homeopathy.* Kluwer Academic Publishers, Dordrecht. p. 65.

Poitevan B, Aubin M, Benveniste J (1986) Approche d'une analyse quantitative de l'effet d'apis mellifica sur la degranulation des basophiles humains in vitro. *Innov. Tech. Biol. Med.* 7: 64. In: Bellavite P and Signorini A (1998) *Fundamental Research in Ultra High Dilution and Homeopathy.* Kluwer Academic Publishers, Dordrecht. p.67.

Poitevan B, Davenas E, Benveniste J (1988) In vitro immunological degranulation of human basophils is modulated by Lung histamine and Apis mellifica. *Brit. J. Clin. Pharmacol.* 25: 439.

Poitevan B (1988) Scientific bases of homeopathy. *Conference at the Société Française des Sciences et Techniques Farmaceutiques.* Bordeaux, France.

Poitevan B (1990) Scientific bases of homeopathy. In: *Homeopathy in Focus.* VGM Verlag fur Ganzheitmedizin, Essen, p. 42.

Popp FA (1986) On the coherence of ultraweak photoemission from living tissues. In: Kilmister C.W. (ed) *Disequilibrium and Self-Organization..* Reidel, Dordrecht. p. 207

Popp FA, Li KH, Gu Q (eds) (1992) *Recent Advances in Biophoton Research.* World Scientific, Singapore.

Projetti ML, Guillemain J, Tetau M (1985) Effets curatifs et préventifs de dilutions homópathiques de sulfate de cuivre appliquées à des racines de lentiles pré- ou post-intoxiquées. *Cahiers de Biothérapie.* **88:** 21–25. Reported in: Schulte J and Endler PC (Eds.) (1998) *Fundamental Research in Ultra High Dilution and Homoeopathy.* The Netherlands: Kluwer Academic Publishers. p. 197.

Reilly DT *et al.* (Oct. 18, 1986) Is Homoeopathy a Placebo Response? Controlled Trial of Homoeopathic Potency, With Pollen in Hayfever as a Model. *The Lancet,* p. 881–885.

Reilly DT *et al.* (1994) Is Evidence for Homoeopathy Reproducible? *The Lancet* **344:** 1601–06

Santini R, Tessier M, Belon P, Pacheco H (1991) Incidence d'un traitement homéopathique par cuprum 4 CH sur le transit intestinal de la souris: etude preliminaire. *C.R. Soc. Biol.* **184:** 55. Reported in: Bellavite P and Signorini A (1995) *Homeopathy: A Frontier in Medical Science.* North Atlantic Books, Berkeley. p. 63.

Schulte J and Endler PC (Eds.) (1998) *Fundamental Research in Ultra High Dilution and Homoeopathy.* The Netherlands: Kluwer Academic Publishers.

Scofield AM (1984) Experimental research in homoeopathy. A critical review (two parts). *Brit. Hom. J.* **73:** 161.

Shaya SY, Smith CW (1977) The effects of magnetic and radiofrequency fields on the activity of lysozyme. *Collective Phenomena* **B:** 215.

Smith CW, Choy R, Monro JA (1985) Water—friend or foe? *Lab. Pract.* **34:** 29.

Smith CW (1988) Electromagnetic effects in humans. In: Frohlich H (ed) *Biological Coherence and Response to External Stimuli.*

Springer-Verlag, Berlin. p. 205

Smith CW (1989) Coherent electromagnetic fields and bio-communication. In: Popp FA *et al* (eds) *Electromagnetic Bio-Information*. Urban and Swarzenberg, München, p. 1.

Smith CW (1994) Electromagnetic and magnetic vector potential bio-information and water. In: Endler PC, Schulte, J (eds) *Ultra High Dilution*. Kluwer Acad. Publ., Dordrecht, p. 187.

Souza Magro I A, *et al.* (1986) Reducao da nefrotoxidade induzida por aminoglucosideos. *41st Liga Medicorum Homoeopathicorum Internationalis Congress,* Rio de Janeiro. Reported in: Schulte J and Endler PC (Eds.) (1998) *Fundamental Research in Ultra High Dilution and Homoeopathy.* The Netherlands: Kluwer Academic Publishers. p. 197.

Sukul NC, Paul A, Sinhababu SP (1993) Hypothalamic neuronal responses of rats to homoeopathic drugs. In: Bornoroni C (ed) *Omeomed92* Editrice Compositori, Bologna. p. 1.

Thiel W, Borho B (1991) Die therapie von frischen, traumatischen Blutergussen der Kniegelenke (Hamartros) mit Traumeel N Injectionslosung. *Biol. Medizin* **20:** 506. Quoted in Bellavite and Signorini (1995), p. 47.

Toper R, Weissman Z, Oberbaum M, Bentwich Z (1990) Effects of high dilutions of antigens on the generation of specific antibodies. In: *Proc. 4th GIRI meeting.* Paris, Abs. 15.

Tsong TY (1989) Deciphering the language of cells. *Trends Biochem. Sci.* **14:**89.

Ullman, D (1994) *Homeopathy: Medicine for the 21st Century.* North Atlantic Books, Berkeley.

Update *US. OTC Market Report.* (July 1994) Essex, England: Nicholas Hall and Co.

Wagner, H (1985) Neue untersuchungen uber die immunostimulierende Wirkung einiger pflanzlicher Homöopathica. *Biologische Medizin* **2:** 399. In: Bellavite P and Signorini A (1998) *Fundamental Research in Ultra High Dilution and Homeopathy.* Kluwer Academic Publishers, Dordrecht. p. 74.

Wagner H, Kreher B, Jurcic K (1988a) In vitro stimulation of human granulocytes and lymphocytes by pico- and femtogram quantities of cytostatic agents. *Arzneimittelforschung Drug Res.* **38**: 273.

Wagner H, Kreher B (1988b) Studi immunologici in vitro e in vivo con farmaci vegetali a bassi dosaggi. *Riv. Ital. Omotossicol.* **VI** (3): 13. In: Bellavite P and Signorini A (1998) *Fundamental Research in Ultra High Dilution and Homeopathy.* Kluwer Academic Publishers, Dordrecht. p. 74.

Wagner H, Kreher B (1989) Cytotoxic agents as immunomodulators. In: *Proceedings of 3rd Meeting of International Group on Very Low Dose Effects.* Atelier Alpha Bleue, Paris, p. 31.

Wiegant FAC, Souren JEM, Van Rijn J, Van Wijk R (1993) Arsenite-induced sensitization and self-tolerance of Reuber H35 hepatoma cells. *Cell. Biol. Toxicol.* 49–59.

Wiegant FAC, Ovelgönne JH, Souren JEM, Van Wijk R (1997a) Stimulation of self-recovery by low doses of arsenite in arsenite-intoxicated cells. In: Bastide (ed). *Signals and Images.* Kluwer Academic Publishers, Dordrecht. pp. 41–51.

Wiegant FAC, Van Rijn J, Van Wijk R (1997b) Enhancement of the stress response by minute amounts of cadmium in sensitized Reuber H35 hepatoma cells. *Toxicology* **116**: 27–37.

Wiegant FAC, Koster D, Nicolai T (1998) A strategy for research into homeopathy. In: Schulte J and Endler PC (Eds.) (1998) *Fundamental Research in Ultra High Dilution and Homoeopathy.* The Netherlands: Kluwer Academic Publishers.

Weisman Z, Topper R, Oberbaum M, Bentwitch Z (1992a) Immunomodulation of specific immune response to KLH by high dilution of antigen. Abstract *GIRI Meeting,* Paris.

Weisman Z, Topper R, Oberbaum M, Harpaz N, Bentwitch Z (1992b) Extremely low doses of antigen can modulate the immune response. *Proc. VIII Intern. Congress Immunol.* Budapest, Hungary, pp. 532.

Williamson AV, Mackie WL, Crawford WJ, Rennie B (1991) A study using Sepia 200c given prophylactically postpartum to prevent anoestrus problems in the dairy cow. *Brit. Hom. J.* 80: 149.

Winston, J (1999) *The Faces of Homeopathy.* Great Auk Publishing. New Zealand.

Wurmser L, Ney J (1955) Mobilisation de l'arsenic fixé chez le cobaye, sous l'action de doses infinitésimales d'arseniate de sodium. *Therapie.* 10: 625.

Youbicier-Simo BJ, Boudard F, Mekaouche M, Bastide M, Bayle JD (1993) Effects of embryonic bursectomy and in ovo administration of highly diluted bursin on adenocorticotropic and immune responses of chickens. *Int. J. Immunother.* 9: 169.

Zell J, Wonnert WD, Mau J, Feuerstake G (1988) Behandlung von akuten Sprunggelenksdistorsionen. Doppelblindstudie zum Wirksamkeitsnachweis eines Homöopatischen Salbenpraparats. *Fortschr. Med.* 106; 96. Quoted in Bellavite and Signorini (1995), p. 47.

Zhou YM, Ho MW, Popp FA, Gu Q (1994) An oscillator cellular automaton model of superdelayed luminescence in synchronously developing populations of early Drosophila embryos. In: Beloussov L, Popp FA (eds) (1998) *Non-Equilibrium and Coherent Systems in Biophysics.* Biology and Biotechnology, Moscow (in press in 1998).

For information in finding a homeopathic practitioner, a newsletter, lay study groups, or training, the best repository of information is:

National Center for Homeopathy
801 Fairfax St., Ste. 306
Alexandria, VA 22314
(703) 548-7790
Fax (703) 548-7792
www.homeopathic.org
nchinfo@igc.org

For contributions to professional training and creation of a teaching clinic, contact:

Homeopathic Patients' Foundation
Linsley Hall
80 Nicholl Ave.
Pt. Richmond, CA 94801
(510) 412-9040

For contributions to further research as described in this book, cost-effectiveness studies, and distance-learning initiatives, call:

Homeopathic Education and Research Organization
(800) 640-8702

About the Author

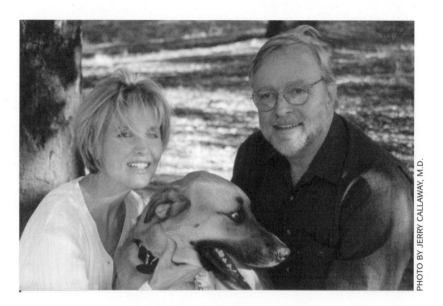

PHOTO BY JERRY CALLAWAY, M.D.

Bill Gray, M.D., has a practice and lives in Saratoga, CA with his artist wife Victoria and their shepherd mix, Bapu.

Dr. Gray graduated from Stanford Medical School in 1970 and began his homeopathic practice in 1971. International lecturer and co-founder of a prestigious homeopathic college, he represented the United States at the Bicentennial Celebration in Frankfurt, Germany, and was the first recipient of the Henry N. Williams Professional Service Award in 1999.

He is also a co-founder of the non-profit Homeopathic Education and Research Organization, which may be reached at (800) 640-8702.